Pr:

Growi

"An unusually intriguing and useful read about how our psychology affects our longevity. If you care about the length and quality of your life but can't stomach yet another diet or workout routine, this book is for you."
—Adam Grant, *New York Times* bestselling author of *Originals* and *Give and Take*, and host of the TED podcast, *WorkLife*

"Finally, a lifestyle book that transcends diet and exercise as solutions for living longer. This well-researched book shows us the subtle power of community and connection as tools for a quest to live to 100."
—Dan Buettner, National Geographic Fellow and *New York Times* bestselling author of *The Blue Zones*

"The more we learn about the human body, the more we realize how powerful the connection between happiness and health is. Research-based, practical, and insightful, *Growing Young* makes this relationship come to life. A must-read."
—Shawn Achor, *New York Times* bestselling author of *Big Potential* and *The Happiness Advantage*

"*Growing Young* is one of the best books I have read on the topic of the mind and its interconnectedness with our body and other human beings."
—Emeran Mayer, author of *The Mind-Gut Connection*

"Friendship is the most important journey we ever venture on. Read Marta Zaraska's *Growing Young* and find out why."
—Robin Dunbar, evolutionary psychologist and author of *How Many Friends Does One Person Need?*

"*Growing Young* is a smart, fresh take on longevity. Deeply researched, fascinating, and engaging, it offers readers useful advice on how to maximize their lifespan, in easy, practical, and unexpected ways."
—Joshua Becker, author of *The More of Less*

"*Growing Young* tells us how to have a long and happy life: Never stop learning and growing. Marta Zaraska's recipes may come from the frontier of research, but it is based on such an elegant distillation of the science that *Growing Young* is as fascinating as it is persuasive."
—Richard Wrangham, professor of biological anthropology at Harvard University and author of *The Goodness Paradox*

"Marta Zaraska's *Growing Young* shows that what matters most is what helps us live the longest! This accessible, well-researched, and thoughtful book is essential reading."
—Greg McKeown, author of the *New York Times* bestselling *Essentialism*

ALSO BY MARTA ZARASKA

Meathooked: The History and Science of
Our 2.5-Million-Year Obsession with Meat

Growing Young

HOW FRIENDSHIP, KINDNESS, AND OPTIMISM CAN HELP YOU LIVE TO 100

Marta Zaraska

appetite

Appetite by Random House® and colophon are registered trademarks of Penguin Random House LLC.

Library and Archives of Canada Cataloguing in Publication is available upon request.

ISBN: 9780525610182
eBook ISBN: 978-525610199

Cover design: Kate Sinclair
Cover image (cake): CSA-Printstock/Getty Images
Printed and bound in the USA

Published in Canada by Appetite by Random House®,
a division of Penguin Random House Canada Limited.

www.penguinrandomhouse.ca

10 9 8 7 6 5 4 3 2 1

appetite
by RANDOM HOUSE

Penguin
Random House
Canada

For Ellie and Maciek—
you've added many years to my life

ACKNOWLEDGEMENTS

WRITING A BOOK CAN BE quite unhealthy at times: the anxiety, the coffee . . . On the other hand, the research for *Growing Young* has connected me with so many kind people I have a feeling that in the end, true to its spirit, it greatly benefited my well-being—and potentially my longevity. I'm particularly grateful to all the scientists who let me into their labs, patiently explaining the nuances of their work: Lynne Cox, with her passion for aging cells and nematode worms; Robin Dunbar, with his unique insights on synchrony (love your office); and Aura Raulo, who let me follow her around the Oxfordshire woods in search of mice while I peppered her with dozens of questions. Carmine Pariante and Naghmeh Nikkheslat— thank you so much for the hours you've spent analyzing my cortisol levels. Without you, my little "experiment" on random kindness and stress levels would not have happened. David Sarphie—learning about leukocyte coping capacity was truly fascinating (and the finger pricking wasn't that bad). Jean-Marie Robine—thank you for enduring the flood of calls and emails about Jeanne Calment. My heartfelt appreciation also goes to the whole Roots of Empathy team, including Christine Zanabi, Cheryl Jackson, and Libby and baby Evelyn— keep doing your amazing work. I'm also deeply indebted to my guide to Japan, Airi Amemiya, who was invaluable in organizing my trip, showing me around Matsudo. Naoki Kondo, Yukiko Uchida, and Shiro Horiuchi helped me navigate the complexities of Japanese culture. Richard Wrangham—thank you for explaining to me how humans self-domesticated. John Gottman—your insights about marriage not only benefited my book, but also my private life.

I'm also grateful to all the people who patiently shared their fascinating stories with me, bringing me a bit closer to understanding the many connections between our mindsets and our health: Lara Aknin—for disclosing her stories on kindness and donations, including the personal ones. Thorbjørn Knudsen—for showing me the extent to which yoga can change us (I'm deeply impressed—and slightly jealous). Vanessa Coggshall—for sharing the bits and pieces of her life with Emmy. Robin Thompson—for opening up about her experiences with shunning. Fujita Masatoshi, Saitou-san, Michiko-san, and Chiaki-san—for letting me experience the great Japanese culture. Katarzyna—for the cuddles. Thank you.

And then there were dozens upon dozens of researchers who generously replied to emails in which I bugged them about their studies as I tried to understand the intricacies of the caregiving system or the HPA axis. Frans de Waal, Boris Bornemann, Fabrizio Benedetti, Larry Young, David Mroczek, John Malouff, Tristen Inagaki, Johan Denollet, Stephen Porges, Rael Cahn, Donald J. Noble, Perla Kaliman, Simon N. Young, Frank Hu, David Steinsaltz, David Sbarra, Janice Kiecolt-Glaser, Thomas Bosch, Kathryn Nelson, Dan Weijers, Kirsten Tillisch, Ed Diener, Paul McAuley, Igor Branchi, Jessica Lakin, and Stefan Schreiber are just a few to whom I'd like to express my gratitude.

Of course, this book would never have happened if it weren't for my lovely and hard-working agent, Martha Webb, as well as for my lovely and hard-working editor, Bhavna Chauhan. Thank you! I'm also grateful to Tom Asker at Little, Brown for believing in *Growing Young* and for introducing it to the British market.

Last but not least, a big, big thank-you to my husband, Maciek, for his unwavering support and enthusiasm, and to my daughter, Ellie, for remaining cheerful even when I shut myself for hours in my office, writing. Each and every day you help me grow young.

CONTENTS

INTRODUCTION

WHEN I WAS A CHILD, besides teaching me how to ride a bike and how to mow the lawn without cutting through the electrical cord, my father taught me the importance of diet and exercise for health and longevity. He instilled in me the importance of eating five veggies a day (and steamed broccoli in particular), the vital role of healthy, unsaturated fats, and the power of phytonutrients found in dark chocolate and red wine. He insisted I play tennis, took me cross-country skiing, and inspired me with his exercise routine—an hour each day, rain or shine. Like any parent, he wants to see me, his child, live to a hundred.

Now that I'm a parent too, I find myself with a similar wish. I want my daughter to one day become a centenarian. What's more, I want to live long enough myself to see her blow out eighty candles on her birthday cake. And so, since the day she was born, I've been fretting over our diets. I mashed organic peas, puréed heritage tomatoes, and froze nutritious soups. In the meantime, I forced myself to eat goji berries and drink kale juice. I encouraged my husband to try fasting and nagged him to go to the gym. I ran a half-marathon. I suffered through thousands of sit-ups.

In the meantime I was writing stories on health and psychology for the *Washington Post, Scientific American,* and many other news outlets. I was digging through hundreds of research papers a year and talking with dozens of scientists. And out of this research a new story began emerging, whether I liked it or not: that my sit-ups and kale juice were not as important to health as I used to think. Intrigued, I delved deeper into the topic. I really wanted to make sure I was doing the best I could to help us all live to a hundred. What I found, repeated over and over in academic papers, shattered my long-held beliefs. Diet and exercise were not the most important things I should be working on to encourage my family's longevity. Instead of shopping for organic goji berries, I should have concentrated on our social lives and psychological makeup. I should have looked for a purpose in life, not the best fitness tracker.

Yet I'm certainly not alone. In our culture we tend to think about longevity in terms of healthy food and exercise. Asked in a poll what they were doing to stay healthy, 56 percent of Americans mentioned "physical activity" and 26 percent "watching food/drink." The only category that might have involved boosting relationships or changing mindsets was "other"—and it got just 8 percent of the vote. We don't realize that volunteering or investing in friendships can help increase our lifespans. Instead, we worry about gluten and obsess about pesticides and mercury in fish. We sign up for Zumba and spinning classes. We search for easy rejuvenating therapies.

The global anti-aging market is already worth upward of $250 billion, and Americans spend more on longevity cures than they do on any other kind of drug, even though most are untested by science. We love pills: about a half of Americans and Canadians take at least one dietary supplement. There are now over 55,000 such products on the US market alone, from moringa leaves to ashwagandha powder. And then, we diet. In one survey, 56 percent of women said they wanted to lose weight to live longer, yet the research on whether this will work is ambiguous. A recent review of almost a hundred studies showed that people who have a BMI (body mass index) of 30 to 35 (that's grade one obesity) are 5 percent less likely to succumb to the grim reaper than those who are lean.

Of course, eating healthy food and doing sports are important for health and longevity, but not as important as we tend to think (and certainly moringa leaves are not required). It's a bit like with smoking and nutrition. Smoking a pack of cigarettes a day is so bad for you that it overshadows the best of diets, but that doesn't mean that non-smokers can rest on their laurels and stuff themselves with junk food. Apart from shunning tobacco, investing in a thriving social life might be the best thing you could do for your longevity. Consider the numbers. Studies show that building a strong support network of family and friends lowers mortality risk by about 45 percent. Exercise, on the other hand, can lower mortality risk by 23 to 33 percent. Eating six or more servings of vegetables and fruits per day, which is admittedly quite a lot, can cut mortality risk by roughly 26 percent, while following the Mediterranean diet—eating lots of fruits, vegetables, and whole grains, replacing butter with olive oil, etc.—21 percent. Of course, such numbers should be taken with caution, coming as they do from studies with varying methodologies, which means they are not straightforward to compare; but they do reveal some important general trends.

The Mediterranean diet has long been touted as the holy grail for those who want to live to a hundred. Just look at my current fellow countrymen, the French: their average lifespan is over four years longer than that of Americans. The longest-lived human ever was French, too. Among Italians, those from Sardinia (a so-called longevity "blue zone") are twenty times as likely as Americans to become centenarians. And so we put the Mediterranean diet under the microscope, analyzing how much cheese the French eat, why skipping breakfast doesn't kill them, and how many grams of fruits they eat each day (and how many of these come in the form of Cabernet). Yet the French don't obsess about the latest dietary fads as much as North Americans or British people do. Along the Seine, gluten doesn't seem to equal evil and neither do carbohydrates.

The French do obsess about their eating—just about a very different aspect of it. Consider my friend's family. For them, not sitting together for dinner, even if it's just an ordinary Monday dinner, is sacrilege. My friend will rush home from our yoga classes and will dash around a supermarket without paying attention to labels (organic? who cares!) just to be on time for the daily dinner ritual. Among the French, 61 percent of those in their thirties and forties eat dinner with their family, at the table, each and every day. Now compare that to the mere 24 percent of Americans that age who do so—and the American data doesn't even specify whether the surveyed people ate together at the table or while watching TV.

What's more, the French, just like the Italians, love their *apéro* (or *aperitivo*, for the Italians). You meet with friends, you drink, you snack. Sometimes you snack so much it's considered dinner—and called *apéro dinatoire*. The French love of apéro is matched only by their love of outings to restaurants—often with the whole family in tow, from kids to grandparents and the family dog. I've even once seen a family bring their horse to a restaurant. It was summer, so they dined outdoors—thankfully. Maybe the life-prolonging aspect of the Mediterranean diet is not the amount of vegetables and olive oil it contains, but the way these foods are eaten—together with others. Maybe it's not what they eat, but how they eat.

In recent years science has begun to unveil how much our minds and bodies are intertwined. Technological advances in molecular biology and brain imaging techniques allow researchers to look deeper into the many links between our thoughts and emotions and our physiology. The vagus nerve, the social hormones oxytocin and serotonin, the stress axes such as the hypothalamic-pituitary-adrenal axis—all of these emerge as the reasons behind why friendships or kindness matter for longevity. Oxytocin, for example, has been linked with our social skills on one hand, and with health on the other. It has anti-inflammatory properties, reduces pain, and helps bone growth, potentially preventing osteoporosis. Studies also show that spraying oxytocin into the nostrils of squabbling married couples makes them more likely to reconcile. It makes us better at reading facial expressions of emotions, and it makes us more trusting. It can even make husbands stand further away from pretty women. Gut microbiota, another link between the body and the mind, play a role in many diseases including diabetes, multiple sclerosis, and allergies, while also affecting emotions and personality. The vagus nerve, the longest of the nerves that emerge directly from the brain, which is responsible for breathing, swallowing, and digestion, has been implicated in sudden psychogenic death reported among the tribes of Africa and the islands of the Pacific.

Some of the discoveries in the field of mind-body connections make it to the media and into the popular culture, yet when it comes to longevity and aging we still seem to prefer a reductionist, strictly biological approach. Take this pill. Eat this superfood. If you do all that, your cells will rejuvenate. It all sounds very authoritative and unambiguous. It's easy to calculate, to the gram, how many leafy vegetables you ate today, how much anti-cancer glucosinolate you ingested with your broccoli, and, thanks to your pedometer, how many steps you took this week. Ray Kurzweil, a futurist, an inventor, and an engineering director at Google, reportedly downs as many as ninety pills a day in an effort to keep himself young.

I fell for the reductionist approach, too. When my six-year-old daughter announced she was going vegetarian, I scoured the internet for the best sources of vitamin B_{12} and iron, calculating to the tenth of a milligram how much she might ingest with every meal. And so I discovered, for instance, that if I had her snack on ten hazelnuts a day that would provide her with 0.48 milligrams of iron. I even started wondering how to add turmeric to every possible recipe—after all, it has an astounding 55 milligrams of iron per 100 grams. Many of us like the safety of numbers, the reassurance of all things quantifiable. From this perspective, the softer psychological and social approaches to longevity may sound a bit confusing. You can't get a friendship-meter to check how well you are doing in terms of your social connections. Are you kind enough? Grateful enough? Is your kid's empathy level sufficient to give them a long and healthy life? After all, empathy does not come in "milligrams per 100 grams" no matter how I wish it did.

In our modern, busy times, it's no wonder that we prefer easily quantifiable longevity quick fixes. Many of us don't have enough hours in a day to focus on all possible things that might influence health. I certainly don't. Between full-time work and taking care of my daughter, there is little time left to think about cardiovascular exercises, organic foods, trying a ketogenic diet, worrying about whether to stop eating gluten, and so on. That is why in this book I prioritize longevity habits and focus on the things that matter the most if you want to live long. Number one? A committed romantic relationship, which according to some studies can lower your mortality risk by a staggering 49 percent. Second, having a large social network of friends, family, and helpful neighbours can reduce the probability of early death by about 45 percent. Third is having a conscientious personality (44 percent).

The benefits brought by the rest of the longevity interventions I describe in this book hover around 20 to 30 percent of mortality risk reduction and play a far greater role in your health than the paleo diet, your turmeric intake, or omega-3 fatty acids (volunteering— about 22 to 44 percent; omega-3s—no effects found). What's more, all these things matter to your centenarian potential at least as much as does a veggie-loaded diet or a busy exercise schedule. Of course, it's a tricky thing trying to compare mortality risks between studies. Studies differ in methodology, the time period when they were conducted, the populations tested (Americans, Japanese, Danish, and so on). I have based my calculations, whenever possible, on the best of studies: meta-analyses and reviews published in respected peer-reviewed journals. Still, the numbers here should be treated as rough guides, not dogma.

To save you time, throughout this book I suggest solutions that marry classic health boosters such as nutrition and physical activity with mental and social efforts. I explain why mowing your elderly neighbour's lawn may be better for your arteries than hitting the gym and why jogging with a friend, in synchrony, could have a higher longevity payoff than running alone (the synchrony is key here). As food goes, rather than gobbling your broccoli without much thought it's more beneficial to eat it mindfully. And for a healthy oxytocin boost, try savouring your greens while looking deeply into your beloved's eyes (research suggests a beloved dog might help, too).

From the perspective of mind-based longevity, becoming a centenarian or raising one often means less work, not more. It means taking a back seat, worrying less, and buying less—fewer toys, fewer fitness gadgets, less organic food. It means letting kids play unsupervised, and letting them get dirty. It means easing up on yourself, spending more time with friends and family, and laughing more often—and the sooner you start, the better.

As I'll argue in this book, besides prioritizing longevity habits we should start working on our mind-based health long before retirement. In one particularly striking study, researchers evaluated aging biomarkers in almost a thousand New Zealanders and found that by the age of thirty-eight some had bodies as young as thirty, while others had a body age as old as fifty—their DNA had deteriorated more rapidly. At thirty or forty, most of us might brood over wrinkles and complain about slow metabolism, but contemplating mortality rates and healthy lifespans doesn't truly take hold until we are deep into our sixties. A recent survey found that the top aging worry for people in their thirties, forties, and fifties was financial security. Yet bad early lifestyle choices can switch genes off and on and erode the telomeres—the caps at the ends of chromosomes that protect our genes from degradation. This, in turn, can mean more life-shortening diseases in later adulthood.

What's worrisome, however, is that in terms of mind-based longevity, young and middle-aged people of today may be worse off than baby boomers. While research continues to underline the power of thought patterns and relationships over our health, polls and surveys bring forward a dark picture: smartphones and social media are destroying our friendships, loneliness is rampant, and empathy levels are plunging. Former president Barack Obama noted that "we live in a culture that discourages empathy." Some policymakers are beginning to take note of these disturbing trends. In 2018 then British prime minister Theresa May appointed a "minister for loneliness" to deal with what she dubbed "the sad reality of modern life," and Manitoba now has a minister responsible for helping seniors stay socially engaged. In the US, Vivek H. Murthy, surgeon general in the Obama administration, went as far as to recognize that loneliness is a health epidemic. He admitted, though, that "many clinicians aren't clear about the strong connection between loneliness and the very health problems we are trying to address, often with medications and procedures." I'm hoping that this book will help raise awareness of these issues, leading to better patient care and health policy decisions.

I wrote *Growing Young* out of a belief that in the deluge of reductionist wellness news we've somehow lost the big picture, ignoring the things that may matter the most for our longevity: relationships, emotions, and the psyche. I'm not a scientist, so I didn't do any of the research personally (other than some "experiments" on myself I conducted for this book). But as a science journalist, I had the freedom to investigate diverse areas of research ranging from molecular biochemistry, epidemiology, neuroscience, zoology, anthropology, psychology, and cyberpsychology to Asian studies, marketing, and so on. I've read over six hundred peer-reviewed academic papers and talked to or corresponded with more than fifty scientists working on the many links between our minds and our health. Admittedly, I also had tons of fun with my research, which took me to unexpected places—catching wild mice in the woods of central England (to check how relationships affect gut microbiota), chatting about Zulu dancing with professor Robin Dunbar in his Hogwarts-like office at Oxford, sipping super-smoothies at a longevity boot camp in Portugal, and arranging flowers with octogenarians in Japan.

After all this research, some of it slightly unpleasant (cortisol swabs), most of it eye-opening, I decided to title this book "Growing Young" to reflect the phenomenon that the very same efforts that rejuvenate our bodies and help us live long also help us grow as people: nurturing relationships, developing better mental habits, becoming kinder, more empathic, more involved in the community. It appears that growing humane grows our centenarian potential.

I've divided this book into two parts. In the first part I explore how we age and how our minds and bodies are interconnected to affect health. In the second part I investigate different psychological and social interventions that affect our longevity—from marriage and friendships to volunteerism and personality changes (yes, it can be done). In each chapter I explain the biological mechanisms and offer practical tips on how to use our mindsets to improve health.

What this book is not, however, is a guide on how to cure diseases with thoughts. The internet is chock-full of claims that you can shrink tumours or heal Lyme disease with positive self-affirmations. These have little base in science. You can't rid yourself of cancer simply by repeating happy phrases in front of a mirror. Even though our mindsets do matter for health and can slow down progress of some illnesses, like Alzheimer's disease for example, there are no secret miracle cures here. Mostly, it's about prevention, just as is the case with healthy diets and exercise.

My goal in writing this book was to help you fundamentally rethink how you approach your health—whether you might be putting too much effort into strategies that don't work well (supplements, fitness trackers, etc.) and not enough into those that truly matter (your love life, your friendships, your life's meaning). But I'm also hoping to entertain you as we discover the roots of Tanganyika's 1962 laughter epidemic, the secrets of booze-loving rodents who mate for life, and why eating undercooked meat might change your personality—with health consequences. We will tour scientific labs from North America and Japan to Siberia, and visit pay-per-hour "huggers" in my birth country, Poland.

Every time I travel to Poland these days to see my dad, he asks me if I take good care of myself. He asks if I eat well, if I exercise, and if I always remember to wear my hat if it's cold outside. I reply, "yes," "yes," and "uhmm . . ." (we don't see eye to eye on the importance of woolly hats for biological well-being). My dad, meanwhile, continues to eat broccoli and swim almost every day despite his advanced age. But besides teaching me the value of phytonutrients and cardio workouts for healthy living, my father has also taught me another valuable lesson. He taught me the importance of constant self-improvement and perseverance. Now, after years of research on the psychological and social roots of longevity, I take his advice a step further: self-improvement, a commitment to growing as a person, can also help us grow younger. That's the core of this book.

PART ONE

THE MIND-BODY CONNECTION
AND ITS LONGEVITY CONSEQUENCES

1

IS DEATH OPTIONAL?

Immortal Animals, Zombie-Killing Pills,
and Super-Centenarians

THE CELL SEEMED BLOATED—its massive, transparent shape filled up half of the microscope's screen. My lab coat crinkled as I leaned closer for a better look: the insides of the cell were cluttered with accumulated "junk"—ripped-up DNA fragments, unwanted proteins, and as many as five nuclei. "It looks immensely old, doesn't it?" Lynne Cox, associate professor of biochemistry at the University of Oxford, nodded toward the giant cell, which, as she told me, came from some guy's foreskin (willingly donated). Turning around, Cox reached into a large incubator to fetch another tray of cells, then popped them under the microscope. The image that appeared was very different from the previous. There were many, many cells on the screen this time, all of them thin, like deflated balloons. "These are from the same guy, just younger cells," she explained, then added, "Aren't they beautiful?"

Cox was my guide for the day to the field of aging. Here in the modern, un-Oxford-like building of the biochemistry department, I got my first look into the scary world of cell senescence and molecular decline. By the first half-hour I was ready to take any miracle longevity pill available (then, fortunately, things got more optimistic).

It may seem obvious that humans age, that with time we get old, wrinkly and liver-spotty. Yet as recently as the eighteenth century people still believed it was possible to live infinitely, or at least well past one thousand. Methuselah made it, supposedly, to 969 years; Zahāk, a figure in Persian mythology, to a thousand; and Tiresias, a Greek prophet, to over six hundred. Even today, while modern science reveals minuscule details about the biochemistry of aging, we are not immune to outrageous longevity claims. Just recently the media picked up the story of an Ecuadorian named Jose David who insisted he was 142 years old, while Mbah Ghoto, an Indonesian, reportedly died in 2017 at the age of 146. It would be great if such feats of the human body were truly possible.

Unfortunately, as one researcher aptly put it, "In our experience, claims to age 130 exist only where records do not." Sometimes birth certificates have been lost or messed up. Sometimes the whole thing is nothing but a case of bad memory. And sometimes it's an outright scam. In Japan, people have been discovered to be collecting pensions for family members who had died decades before.

In reality, basically all supercentenarians, or people who live beyond 110, pass away around their 115th birthdays. The record for the US is currently 119, for Canada 117, for Spain 114, for Germany 112, and so on. Which raises the question: Is there some kind of natural limit to the human lifespan? If you take two longevity researchers and ask them about such a limit, chances are a fight will ensue. When in 2016 several scientists published a paper claiming that the maximum human lifespan fluctuates around 115, the back and forth of yeas and nays was astounding. Many said the analysis was accurate. Others claimed it to be flawed, full of erroneous assumptions (mostly math-related). In this study, as in several others in which scientists tried to calculate the human age limit, one problem kept popping up which, according to some researchers, skewed the results. That problem's name was Jeanne Calment.

Why the Universe Doesn't Care about Old People

The first time Jean-Marie Robine entered what he now calls "that awful nursing home," a big concrete building straight out of the 1970s located in Arles, France, he expected to meet there a feeble-minded old lady, blind and deaf, with whom he wouldn't be able to communicate. After all, she was already 117 years old at the time. Yet the moment he swung open the doors to her room he realized he was in for a surprise. Jeanne Calment greeted him with a strong and very conscious "*Bonjour, monsieur.*" She might have been old, but she wasn't feeble.

Robine, a gerontologist at INSERM, the French National Institute of Health and Medical Research, "found" Calment when he and his colleagues were gathering profiles of French centenarians back in the early 1990s. At first, they put her survey aside, worried that such an outlier would just mess up the data. "We said: what can we do with a person 115 years old? We were interested in centenarians, not people fifteen years later!" Robine tells me.

In the meantime, Calment was also "discovered" by a Canadian movie crew that was working on a film about Vincent van Gogh. Someone in Arles, Van Gogh's hometown, told the Canadians that there was still a woman living there who had met the painter. They found her, and she confirmed that she indeed had known Van Gogh—which Robine is not convinced was the truth (some dates just don't add up, he says). But once *Vincent and Me* hit the screens, Calment became a star. Not only was Calment, at 115, officially the oldest actress in history, she was also one of the oldest people to have ever walked the earth. The press was all over her.

Calment turned 116. Then 117. And Robine decided it was time to have a look at that file of hers. Her unusually old age intrigued him, so he set up a meeting in the nursing home. Since that day he has met her about forty times and researched her case extensively.

Calment ended up setting a record for human longevity—she made it to 122 years and 164 days—which, in case you are wondering, has been verified and established beyond doubt. Yet whenever Robine asked her if she had any ideas for what might have caused her to live that long, she would just shrug and say that God had forgotten her. That's unusual, since in Robine's experience, centenarians usually like to offer plenty of explanations for their endurance. "We had about 900 centenarians in our survey, and they gave us on average more than one longevity secret. They were all over the place. One centenarian would say: 'I started working when I was 14 and I've never stopped. That's my secret.' Then another would say: 'I've never worked in my life—that's my secret.' So basically there was no secret," Robine says.

Calment liked to amaze journalists, whom she adored, with tales of her cigarette smoking and port wine drinking. But these were lies, too, Robine tells me. She only smoked for about two years (starting well after her 110th birthday), and only smoked one Gauloise per night, as a social thing to share with a smoker friend. She admitted to Robine that she would tell the media whatever they liked to hear, and a cigarette-puffing, boozing centenarian does make for a good story. Even the *New York Times* fell for it, reporting in her obituary that she "only quit smoking five years ago."

Robine believes that the lies and the love of interviews revealed something important about Calment's personality, and possibly some part of her longevity secret. She was strong, rebellious, curious about the world, and fiercely independent. As a child and a young woman she was supposedly so out of control that her father would not allow her to go anywhere unsupervised. As a married woman, Calment loved to try new things: helicopter flights, skiing, you name it—and remember that we are talking about the late nineteenth and early twentieth century here. One of the first things she did after getting married, even before the wedding night, was to ask her husband for a cigarette so that she could finally experience smoking (her father hadn't allowed it). She took a puff and then extinguished the cigarette right away. She had tried it; that was all she wanted. She loved savouring all life had to offer.

She was happy with her husband, Ferdinand. They were married for almost half a century, and she would later claim that she only had good memories of their time together. She'd say he was the "perfect man," Robine tells me, and she never tried to remarry after his death. Ferdinand was seven years older than Jeanne, and died in 1942 at the age of seventy-three.

When Calment agreed to be moved to a nursing home at the age of 110 (after she had almost set her house on fire by trying to defrost the pipes with a self-made torch—long story), she made three demands: that the staff would provide a hotel-style bed turndown service for her; that every day she would be woken up fifteen minutes before everyone else so that she had time to primp herself; and that the head doctor would allow her to call him "my dear." Yes, she was bossy. But above all, she was an optimist, something that Robine speculates was at least in part responsible for her longevity. Calment divided life's events into two groups, he tells me. First: things you could change. These you should act on right away. Second: things you couldn't change. These you should forget.

It may seem unbelievable that Jeanne Calment enjoyed relatively good health until the very end. In reality, though, that was to be expected. Here is some surprising biology: studies show that the longer you live, the higher the likelihood of staying in close-to-perfect shape until the day you drop dead while gardening or roller-blading across the globe. We tend to be amazed by media stories of centenarians jumping with parachutes or participating in marathons. We shouldn't be. In a way, it's less remarkable that a centenarian can run long-distance than an eighty-year-old. While a regular Joe or Sue will spend almost 18 percent of their time on earth overtaken by disease—admittedly not a happy prospect—for an average supercentenarian that number is just 5 percent. Typically, they stay in good health until the age of 109, and one in ten manages to escape disease till the very last three months of their lives.

When I read these numbers, my first thought was that such people must have some remarkable genes (something I probably don't possess). Research indicates that there may be some truth to this. Calment's personality alone likely wouldn't have been enough to push her over the 115-birthday threshold. She probably had the genes for it, too. Robine and his colleagues managed to find the length-of-life data for fifty-five direct ancestors of Calment, spanning five generations all the way back to the seventeenth century. They also created a control "family" by including individuals of the same sex married in the same municipality as Calment's ancestors and who appeared on the register of marriages just before or just after them. This way they discovered an unprecedented number of long-lived people in Calment's family: as many as thirteen out of the fifty-five lived to be over eighty years old, an achievement in the seventeenth and eighteenth centuries. In the control "family" only one person lived that long. That's 24 percent versus 2 percent.

Robine now believes that Calment did indeed have an unusual accumulation of good genes. Still, she was an outlier. For most of us, how long we live is only about 20 to 25 percent heritable. What's more, although scientists have been on the lookout for specific longevity genes for quite some time now, the results are less than impressive. There appear to be plenty of different genes associated with lifespan—we have discovered over a hundred of them in mice alone. It's impossible to tell at this point which particular genes might have helped Calment live as long as she did. Hopefully we will know more in the future, since a vial of Calment's blood, with all the precious information in it, is still held in one lab in Paris.

Although Calment's case certainly stretched our knowledge about how long humans can live, it did little to answer another question that keeps bugging researchers: whether aging itself is unavoidable. Until very recently, it seemed that it was. And then came the hydra.

A typical freshwater hydra is usually under 0.39 inches (1 cm) long, so to see it well you have to put it under a microscope. It has a head with long tentacles and a tube-like body, reminding me of Sideshow Bob from *The Simpsons*. And just like Sideshow Bob, hydras are immortal—at least as long as they are kept in the relative safety of a lab, since in the wild they tend to succumb to various accidents in a matter of weeks. If kept in petri dishes, away from predators and other environmental dangers, these animals have such amazingly low mortality rates that many would be still alive after three thousand years (even in labs accidental deaths happen, like when a researcher forgets to close a hydra-containing dish properly and the hydras dry out—true story).

From the fact that hydras can live forever, we now know that aging can be side-stepped. Why does it exist at all in the first place, then? Is it part of nature's programmed plan? Or is it just an unpleasant side effect of living? These, too, are questions that tend to put many scientists on edge, with some voting for the aging-is-programmed theory and others—admittedly, the majority—favouring the view that we get old simply because the universe doesn't care much about what happens to you once you've passed on your genes.

The thing is that some of the genes that are very beneficial when your goal is to make tons of babies have detrimental side effects down the road, once you've stopped reproducing. Take the genes encoding the growth hormone that on the one hand boosts fertility, but on the other hand accelerates aging and promotes cancer. Natural selection doesn't really act once your gene-passing—that is, baby-making—times are over, so there is no selection pressure to wipe out genes that have harmful effects later in life. In case you are into names, this theory has a complicated one: "antagonistic pleiotropy"—basically meaning "opposing effects" (good when young, bad when old). Antagonistic pleiotropy is likely one reason mice have shorter lives than elephants. If you are a tiny vermin, you have to reproduce fast before you get snatched by a cat or a snake. You breed, you deteriorate, you die. But massive elephants, with low risk of accidental death, can take their time awaiting offspring—and as a result can reach the age of sixty years or more.

As we get older, our bodies slowly fall apart due to simple wear and tear, which, from an evolutionary perspective, is not worth cleaning up. We accumulate mutations and damage to our DNA, mitochondria, and proteins. And if you want to see how this damage works in practice, there is hardly a better creature to observe than the tiny worm *Caenorhabditis elegans*, or *C. elegans* for short.

Old Mitochondria, Telomeres, and Longevity Genes

"Is it dead?" I asked as I stared down the microscope at a minuscule creature that resembles an earthworm. The animal hadn't moved in what felt like forever.

"Nah, just old," Lynne Cox replied as she took a look through the eyepiece herself. "It must be on its last legs, though. Can you see how the insides are all shrivelled up? Although it's not as wrinkly as they can get," Cox said, then chuckled. "It aged well—maybe this one here is an optimistic worm?" I watched as she changed the dish under the microscope for a different one, glass scraping against the plastic. In a white-walled lab cluttered with black-and-white equipment, the purple gloves on Cox's hands stood out in a splash of colour. The air smelled of latex and disinfectant. Done with the dish swap, the biochemist encouraged me to check out the contents of the new one. I looked down. Now there was plenty of movement on the little glass. Dozens of *C. elegans* were squirming in a snake-like fashion, wriggling around. These guys were barely five days old—the equivalent of humans in their twenties. "Can you see how they are moving happily?" Cox asked me. She sighed. "They are cool, aren't they? You tend to fall in love with these worms when you work with them."

Longevity researchers do indeed have plenty of reasons to fall in love with *C. elegans*. The worms are ultra-easy to breed, they share a large amount of their genome with humans, most of them are hermaphrodites—so each can reproduce on its own, making tons of genetically identical copies—and, on top of everything, they are see-through. With just a glimpse through a microscope you can observe all the changes happening in the worms' bodies without the need to cut them open. "As they age you can see the whole structure of the tissues break down," Cox told me. What's more, if you want to change their gene expression, all you have to do is feed them specially prepared bacteria. It's no wonder then that Cox and her colleagues chose *C. elegans* to study the changes that aging inflicts on a molecular level, including damage to the DNA.

Just like in *C. elegans*, almost all of your cells contain DNA—long, two-stranded molecules, most of it inside the nucleus, and a tiny bit in the mitochondria, the cells' powerhouses. But your DNA doesn't stay unchanged throughout your life. Much the same as your favourite shoes or the book you've read many times, DNA gets worn out with use. Sometimes it's outside factors, such as radiation or chemicals, that can cause mutations. Or it can be due to simple mistakes during cell replication. And sometimes the damage is done by free radicals, by-products of energy production inside the cell. As a result, the DNA strands can get small lesions or even break completely. Most of the time, the cell's cleaning and repair services will march in and fix the problem. But like any mechanic, these processes are not perfect, and will overlook some of the damage or make additional mistakes. Year after year, the flaws in your DNA will accumulate. This, in turn, can lead to such health problems as cancer, cardiovascular issues, and Alzheimer's disease.

The DNA in your cells' mitochondria, the free radical–producing powerhouse, can get damaged even more than that in the nucleus (imagine keeping your favourite book beside an open fire). Other stuff in the mitochondria suffers, too: the membranes, the proteins, the lipids. With time, the mitochondria decline in function—they simply stop producing enough energy to power the cell. That's one of the main reasons why the old, wrinkly *C. elegans* I observed under Cox's microscope barely moved. That may also be part of the reason why by 5 p.m. I'm usually ready to plop down tiredly on the couch while my six-year-old daughter keeps jumping around like a bouncy rabbit, as if showing off the power of her young, undamaged mitochondria.

Some ancient philosophers used to believe that we die because each person is born with a limited number of breaths or heartbeats that we can have in life. When you use them up, you kick the bucket. Modern science shows that there may be something to this way of thinking, although it's not breaths or heartbeats that are finite (of course). What we run out of are pairs of telomeres—parts of the DNA that function as protective caps at the ends of chromosomes, and which are often compared to aglets—those plastic thingies on shoelaces that prevent fraying.

When you are born you have about ten thousand base pairs of DNA making up the telomeres on each of your chromosomes. But every time a cell in your body divides, you lose anywhere from fifty to two hundred of those pairs. What's more, just like any part of the DNA, telomeres can get damaged by free radicals. And once they get too short, the cell may stop dividing and even die. That, in turn, has been linked to aging.

If you are into books and articles on longevity, and have read a few in the recent past, you probably have already come across telomeres—they feature quite prominently in many such publications, often paired with expressions such as "miracle," "immortality," or "key to longevity." Just eat this and that, the thinking goes, exercise X minutes a day, and your telomeres will stay long, which in turn will make you stay young.

The first time I read about telomeres I was quite excited: here was an easy way to measure aging and anti-aging therapies. But as I dug deeper into new research, my hopes dispersed. It seems that the role of telomeres in aging has been quite overhyped. Cox goes as far as to say that the telomere field "worries her a bit." The early thinking was that telomeres could act as a kind of a biological clock: since we lose about twenty-five base pairs per year, you could assume that someone who had shorter telomeres was biologically older than someone with long telomeres, irrespective of what their birth certificate said. Thanks to recent studies, however, we now know that the biggest difference in telomere length between any two people is already apparent at birth. Some of us are simply born with hundreds of extra pairs. Part of the reason is genetics. Another is your mom (yes, you can blame her now). "Suboptimal intrauterine conditions," as scientists call it, basically refers to things such as maternal stress, smoking, bad diet, and exposure to air pollution, all of which have been shown to considerably shorten the telomeres of babies.

Yet having shorter telomeres is not always that bad. In fact, in line with the antagonistic pleiotropy theory, short telomeres can protect animals from developing cancer, especially in youth. Considering their size, elephants should have about a million-fold higher risk of cancer than your average mouse (the more cells you have, the greater the chances that some of them will go rogue). And yet, elephants don't get much cancer. Most likely, they are protected by their short telomeres and a subdued activity of an enzyme called telomerase that can extend the telomeres.

The telomerase-cancer link, which has also been shown in humans, is among the reasons Cox is so weary of the media hype surrounding telomeres. On the internet you can now purchase supplements claimed to activate telomerase, promising "anti-aging from the inside out" or reduction in "cellular aging." If you take telomerase pills you could, maybe, roll back the speed of your aging—although even that is speculative—but the side effect might be cancer. As it often is in biology, telomeres are about balance, keeping in check cancer versus degenerative diseases, and oversimplifications may be dangerous.

A better biological aging clock, many scientists now argue, is based on DNA methylation, also known as the "epigenetic clock." As we get older, our cells collect more and more epigenetic changes—changes that turn genes on or off without affecting the DNA sequence itself. Your diet, stress levels, whether you meditate—all this can speed up or slow down your epigenetic clock, leaving visible marks in the appearance of your DNA for scientists to analyze. Unsurprisingly, some commercial labs are already offering to measure your epigenetic clock. Pay a few hundred dollars, send in a blood sample, and you will receive an estimation of your DNA methylation age. Studies show that for about half of people, their epigenetic age differs only by less than 3.6 years from their chronological age, but for some others the difference is astounding: some forty-year-olds have a DNA methylation age as low as twenty, while others have one as high as fifty. That's a three-decade spread!

What links epigenetic changes, telomere shortening, DNA damage, and damage to other parts of the cell such as mitochondria, proteins, and lipids, is that these are all involved in something that scientists call "cellular senescence"—or in simpler words, cellular aging, a phenomenon that makes cells fat, useless, and full of junk, just like the one I saw in Cox's lab. A healthy young cell is a cell that grows and divides. If it's useless or too damaged, it commits suicide. That's how your tissues—like your skin, for instance—get renewed. But sometimes a cell that has accumulated a lot of damage stops dividing, but doesn't kill itself either. It just sits there, getting bigger and bigger, collecting whole piles of waste, such as misfolded proteins and old mitochondria.

"Normally if your mitochondria stop working you digest them down and make new ones. But old cells just keep their damaged mitochondria—they fill up, like garbage cans. That's one of the reasons the old cells are so huge," Cox tells me. Such bloated senescent cells are not quite dead. And these zombie cells accumulate as we age, belching out toxins called senescence-associated secretory phenotype, which in true zombie style can turn other cells senescent, too. What makes things even worse is that the secretions from senescent cells promote low-level chronic inflammation that is sometimes called "inflammaging," and which lies at the basis of most age-related diseases such as Alzheimer's disease, rheumatoid arthritis, diabetes, cancer, and heart disease.

Can't we then just go in with some drugs and kill all the zombie cells, I wondered? Go *World War Z* on them? It could potentially work. In animal studies, destroying senescent cells delays aging and even prolongs lifespans by about 25 percent (imagine living ninety-seven years instead of the current American average of seventy-eight). Senolytics, drugs that kill zombie cells, and which are ready for clinical trials, are touted by some as the potential anti-aging cure. But there are a few problems with them, I soon learned. First of all, there are potential side effects, such as delayed wound healing. Second, what works in rats doesn't necessarily work in humans. Cox is also cautious. "If you have lots of senescent cells, you can't kill, say, 75 percent of your body. And if you suddenly find out that the drugs are taking out too many cells in one go, what do you do?" she asks.

If any animals do not need senolytics, it's certainly the hydras, the immortal Sideshow Bob look-alikes. When scientists tracked generations of offspring of individual cells taken from the gastric region of hydras, they discovered that they simply don't turn into zombies. It makes sense: most cells of the hydras are stem cells, which never stop proliferating, constantly renewing the bodies of these tiny creatures. The reason for this, and in effect for the hydras' immortality, is the way they breed. Instead of having males mate with females, hydras make babies asexually by budding. To reproduce, they need a constant and reliable supply of freshly divided cells.

Although we will likely never achieve hydra-like immortality (our bodies are far more complicated than theirs), we can certainly learn a few things about aging from the workings of hydras' stem cells. Stem cells—whether hydra or human ones—are quite amazing little things. They are created shortly after fertilization and then go on to make new, specialized cells throughout our lives, helping us grow and renew tissues. Yet stem cells are not immune to damage, either. As years pass, our stem cells work less and less well, go "zombie," or die, and their numbers diminish, a process which has been implicated as one of the top reasons for aging.

At least for humans. Hydras are particularly good at repair and maintenance of their stem cells. One type of genes, called *FOXOs* (otherwise known as the forkhead box O; a lot of genes have strange names) may play a role in this and could be quite important for longevity, from hydras and mice to whales and Jeanne Calment. These particular genes work to protect cells from damage and are involved in DNA repair. In hydras, *FOXOs* keep stem cells going. If you reduce the activity of *FOXOs* in these tiny creatures, they turn mortal. In humans, a particular sequence variation in one type of *FOXO* gene, *FOXO3a*, has been linked to longevity in various populations, from American men of Japanese ancestry to the Chinese and Germans.

But don't rush to the internet to look for a lab that will check your *FOXO3a* polymorphisms. We are much more complicated creatures than hydras; most likely, *FOXO3a* is just one among many genes responsible for why some people live longer than others (and anyway, longevity is just 20 to 25 percent heritable, remember?).

Women Ahead

That women and men differ in terms of longevity is certainly not news to anyone. Just take a stroll through your local graveyard. My grandma keeps joking that Grandpa likes to visit the graves of our relatives so that he can flirt with all these widows he meets at the cemetery. After all, he is a rare sight there: a Polish gentleman in his late eighties. Admittedly, Poland has quite a large spread between the female and male life expectancies—it's eighty-one for women and seventy-three for men. Lithuania is even worse, with a ten-year gap, and Russia tops the world's charts with 11.6 years of difference between the sexes (the male penchant for vodka certainly plays a role). On the other end of the scale are countries such as Iceland (a 3.0 year gap in favour of women), Sweden (3.4 years), or the UK (3.6 years). Curiously, in the past, men and women could look ahead to living for a comparable amount of time. In the 1800s in Sweden the life expectancy at birth was thirty-three years for women and thirty-one years for men, and other places were likely similar. Fate simply cut everyone's existence short: birthing kids, infections, and wars.

Once birthing kids, infections, and wars stopped flattening the playing field for everyone, however, the gap between men and women widened, reaching its largest between the 1970s and 1990s. Nowadays, with men starting to take better care of themselves, they are once again catching up—but not quite. Somehow women always seem ahead in terms of longevity, whether we are talking nineteenth-century Scandinavia or contemporary India or Canada. What's going on, then? Is it still all due to healthier female lifestyles? Less gun-shooting, less show-off driving, and more broccoli? Not exactly. Scientists now believe that the female-male longevity gap is actually imprinted into our bodies, and one of the clues comes from how women and men survive catastrophic conditions.

On the night of November 3, 1846, heavy snow coated the eastern slopes of the Sierra Nevada. A group of Midwestern farmers and businessmen, their wives, children, and family pets in tow, got stranded around Truckee Lake (later renamed Donner Lake), a large, whale-shaped body of water at the foot of the mountains. In the morning of November 4, the eighty-one members of the group woke up surrounded by ten-foot-high drifts of snow. Impassable.

The Donner party, as it is now known after the name of their leader, George Donner, had set off from their homes in the Mississippi valley in search of a better life in California. But they'd made a mistake. Instead of taking the usual route through present-day Idaho, they chose what was supposed to be a shortcut crossing the Great Salt Lake Desert. The shortcut proved harder than the original route. The group didn't make it in time to cross the Sierra Nevada before winter. With the new, heavy snow, they were stuck.

Cut off from the world, with dwindling food supplies and close to no outdoor skills, the Donner party started suffering "maniacal cravings for food." They ate their dogs. They cooked animal hides into jelly they could swallow. And by February they began eating their own dead. Once the rescue finally came, thirty-five out of eighty-one had died, by and large from hunger and hypothermia. Curiously, most of the dead were men.

Researchers have calculated that among the Donner party, the male mortality risk was almost double the female one. They attributed this to the fact that women in general tend to survive starvation better, which came up in data from many historical famines, including the Ukrainian famine of 1933 and the Irish one of 1845 to 1849. The reason for this, scientists argue, is that women tend to be smaller than men, have a lower basal metabolic rate and a larger proportion of subcutaneous fat—the jiggly type right under the skin. This allows them to survive on less food, while the fat keeps them warm. It's ironic that the very thing that's the bane of so many women's existence (belly fat!) is the same thing that's keeping them alive over men.

Although in the modern-day West starvation is rarely an issue, men still live shorter lives than do women, even in strictly controlled conditions. When German researchers looked at over eleven thousand Catholic nuns and monks from Bavarian cloisters, they discovered that there still remained about a year of difference in favour of the sisters. Females of other mammal species, from chimpanzees and lions to American beavers and European rabbits, have a similar advantage. In a comparison of fifty-nine species inhabiting zoos, only four had males that outlived the females. Certainly smoking and vodka were not to blame.

One key to the mystery of the male-female longevity gap may lie in our chromosomes. Since women have two X chromosomes, they basically have a spare copy of every gene in their bodies to replace a defective one in case of need. Second, women tend to be shorter than men, so they have fewer cells to go awry in the first place (it's like with mice and elephants and their million-fold higher cancer risk). Yet another hypothesis suggests that because each woman's heart rate goes up during the second half of the menstrual cycle, their tickers get exercised in a similar way to how joggers exercise theirs—which could explain why women tend to get cardiovascular disease later in life than men do.

And then, there are the hormones. An analysis of lifespans of eunuchs living in nineteenth-century Korean courts revealed that they survived on average twenty years longer than did other men in the court, including the kings. What eunuchs are short on, of course, is testosterone, which, studies show, tends to suppress the immune system, making men more susceptible to viruses and bacteria. On the other hand, female hormones such as estrogens give a boost to the immune system while also helping the cleanup of bad cholesterol from the arteries.

Since cutting off their male parts does not seem to appeal to most contemporary men, a search for other potential boosts to longevity is in full swing. In a way, that's nothing new—conquistador Ponce de León supposedly hunted for the fountain of youth way back in the sixteenth century. Yet these days the search happens mostly in biotech labs, and its focus is on pills and injections, not magic water sources.

Magic Pills and Plasma Infusions

In an interview for *The New Yorker* back in 2017, the futurist Ray Kurzweil admitted to downing as many as ninety pills a day in an effort to keep himself young and boost his centenarian potential. One of these pills was metformin, a diabetes drug which, Cox tells me, is currently taken by nearly everybody she knows from the US who is working on aging. There is growing evidence that metformin may indeed prolong life and delay aging—it does so in mice and in *C. elegans*. At a cellular level it reduces production of reactive oxygen species and decreases DNA damage (among other effects). But Cox herself does not take metformin. "Any pharmaceuticals will have side effects. And we don't really know the long-term effects of metformin in people who don't have a clinical need to take it," she says.

Many of the therapies currently hyped in Silicon Valley as the next fountain of youth haven't undergone rigorous testing on humans and are, at best, just "promising." A molecule called NAD+, which could potentially rejuvenate the mitochondria, was just entering clinical trials at the time of writing. Rapamycin, an immunosuppressant commonly used to prevent rejection of transplanted organs, could help regulate cellular suicide and growth—but there are already reports of serious side effects including toxicity to kidneys and decreases in blood platelets.

Other proposed longevity therapies are even more disturbing. You could, for instance, get an infusion of blood from a younger person. In rather creepy experiments, scientists sewed together the circulatory systems of two rats, an old one and a young one, so that the elderly rodent would get an infusion of young blood, and discovered that this boosted the senior's lifespan. Some companies in the US are already preparing to run clinical trials on elderly humans (don't worry, no one will sew them to teenagers—it would be done by blood transfusions). But many scientists are wary of the whole idea. In an interview for *Scientific American*, one University of California molecular biologist said it "just reeks of snake oil." To me, it brought to mind a warning Stephen Colbert gave to American youth on *The Late Show*: that President Trump was going to replace Obamacare with mandatory blood exchanges from teens to rejuvenate the aging population: "He's going to stick a straw in you like a Capri-Sun," he said.

If vampire-style longevity remedies don't appeal to you, you could always go for stem cell treatments instead. Several biotech companies in North America now offer banking of stem cells derived from a variety of sources, including umbilical cord blood, menstrual blood, and baby teeth. The hope here is that we will be able to use these cells to rejuvenate tissues. Yet stem cell therapies are still in infancy. At best, their anti-aging effects are just uncertain. At worst, they may be dangerous. When one Florida company tried to treat age-related macular degeneration with stem cells, three women ended up blind.

When I think of a longevity pill, the idea seems really appealing at first. No need to exercise, eat well, or take care of my social life. Just swallow and be young forever, my mitochondria rejuvenating, my DNA fixing itself, my proteins folding correctly. If all promises of stem cells, senolytics, and organ replacements pan out, maybe some of us could become immortal, regenerating over and over. Many in Silicon Valley are certainly banking on that. But assuming hydra-like immortality is attainable for humans, would pursuing it actually be a good idea? First of all, if we were immortal, our lives could lose their meaning. Nothing would matter anymore if you had all the time in the world to get anything you wanted. One study, aptly titled "The Scrooge Effect," revealed in a series of experiments that people derive more pleasure from donating money if they are reminded of their own mortality. How much pleasure in living would we lose by living forever?

Then there is the ethical side of the immortality question. Around the world there are children dying of starvation by the thousands—should we really be spending so much research money on finding some miraculous longevity pill? Our planet is already overpopulated and its resources stretched to the limit. How many immortal humans could the earth withstand? Certainly not everyone that is born, right? So how do we pick who lives forever and who degenerates and dies? And what if immortality or extreme longevity was indeed achievable, and dictators could stay in power in perpetuity? Imagine if Stalin never died or Castro never aged.

A better idea than chasing the holy grail of ridiculously long life-spans may be focusing on something far more attainable: prolong-ing average health-spans, which usually has the neat side effect of upping our chances of becoming centenarians anyway. Instead of the few wealthiest one-percenters living to 150 or 200, we could have societies where many reach their hundredth birthdays in good health. We know from research on supercentenarians that the longer people live, the longer they tend to stay in good shape. Instead of occupying hospital beds and draining health care budgets, these seniors would still be productive members of the community. Giving instead of taking. And, of course, suffering less, too.

Ethical questions aside, we are unlikely to discover one magic longevity pill any time soon. Our bodies are complicated, far more so than those of hydras, *C. elegans*, or mice. What works for rodents won't necessarily work for humans. And then there are the potential side effects to consider. Metformin, for instance, has been shown to cause diarrhea, cold sweats, coma, seizures, and racing heartbeat.

There are no easy fixes no matter how much we would love them, so instead of hoping for the fountain of youth, we should embrace solutions that do work. Eating right, exercising, and above all, taking care of our minds and social lives. Changing our mindsets, not our medicine cabinets. Living in a community where neighbours care about one another means, for women, cutting the risk of coronary heart disease by a third. Chronic loneliness, on the other hand, can up your mortality risk by 83 percent—which is worse than cigarettes. Longevity pills may be tempting, but volunteering or improving friendships won't give you seizures or a racing heartbeat (unless we are talking romantic friendships, that is).

Jeanne Calment might have lived long due to her genes, but perhaps also due to her have-no-regrets personality. Optimism can prolong life by as much as ten years, while lack of rumination on past mishaps boosts the immune system in the elderly. What's more, Calment was happily married for decades, and studies shows that married people live longer, are more likely to survive heart attacks, and even respond better to flu vaccines. For cancer, marriage may be sometimes better than chemotherapy.

Jeanne Calment may have also gained a year or two simply by being a woman—perhaps because of her double X chromosomes, but maybe also because women tend to be more empathic and socially integrated, which helps longevity, too (more on that in chapters 6 and 7). Such links between sociality and health are hardly surprising. After all, our bodies and minds are connected in myriad ways: through our stress axes, our immune systems, and even the three pounds of microbes that reside in our guts.

A FEW SUGGESTIONS TO BOOST YOUR LONGEVITY

Don't trust anyone who tells you they've discovered a secret to longevity.

Don't waste your money on genetic predict-your-lifespan tests or banking your own stem cells—their efficacy is doubtful at best. Don't obsess about your telomeres. If you do have a few hundred spare dollars, and really want to test something, measure your epigenetic clock. Forget miracle longevity pills—many of them are simply dangerous. If you want to live longer, try to find a romantic partner or work on your current relationship—being happily married can lower your mortality risk even by 49 percent. Or volunteer, which may lower your risk of death by about 22 percent.

HOW YOUR MIND TALKS
WITH YOUR BODY

Mortgage Worries, Stress-Resistant Nazis,
and a Few Trillion Microbes

IN THE 1979 MOVIE *Manhattan* Diane Keaton asks Woody Allen to let out his anger so that they can finally get things "out in the open." "I don't get angry," he replies, "I grow a tumour instead."

Woody Allen might have been on to something. Our bodies and minds are amazingly interconnected. In experiments, people who merely imagine exercising their hand muscles end up with improved strength. Others get real rashes from exposure to fake poison ivy. Placebo treatments, meanwhile, are so effective that 42 percent of balding men maintain or increase hair growth after such "cures." Hypnosis can even be used to reduce pain during lumbar punctures and heart surgeries.

There is nothing magical or New Agey about body-mind connections. Instead, very measurable neural, hormonal, and immunological pathways link our thoughts and feelings to other physiological processes in our bodies. William Paul Young, a Canadian novelist, once wrote that "emotions are the colors of the soul"—a sublime statement, but rubbish from the perspective of modern biology. Emotions are not fairy-dust clouds floating around in our heads. They are evolved signals inside the body that exist as much in humans as they do in other animals, from cows and dogs to birds and reptiles.

If you take an animal and apply electrical stimulation to its brain-stem, that ancient structure at the base of the brain, you will elicit behaviours suggestive of emotions. The same thing works with humans too, indicating that emotions are very old in evolutionary terms and that besides inspiring poetry they must serve some very down-to-earth purposes, like helping you not get eaten by preda-tors. Emotions inform us about the state of our environment and our bodies and help us prepare an adequate response. Fear? A lion may be approaching. Anger? You may soon get punched. Disgust? Don't touch! Parasites could be lurking. Satisfaction? All is well in your body.

Emotions may also facilitate learning—things that are emotion-ally loaded simply get better ingrained in our memory. You may well remember to avoid nighttime strolls through the savanna if you were once scared there by a predator. In lab experiments, people are best at recalling memories that are emotionally intense, regard-less how much time has passed since the experience. The idea that emotions serve as guides to bodily sensations and the environment is further supported by the fact that people paralyzed from the neck down often complain that their emotions are blunted.

Of course, even if lizards and ducks do have emotions, our inner lives are likely more complicated than are theirs. That's why neuro-scientists tend to distinguish emotions from feelings, the latter being the mental experiences of emotions—yet still very much planted in our biology (the cerebral cortex is involved). Emotion is basically that thing that stirs in your gut or your chest. Feeling is what your brain does with that stir, how it experiences it. Emotions are our guide to the environment. Feelings are how we interpret the signs. Emotions are automatic, while feelings are more conscious.

Just like emotions and feelings, our thoughts aren't ethereal vapours, either. Researchers are still arguing over where exactly in the brain self-generated thoughts arise, but some patterns are beginning to emerge. A region called the default network seems particularly vital—that's a network of brain regions that activates when you are not doing anything in particular, kind of like a computer on standby.

If you wonder how, exactly, scientists find thoughts inside human skulls, here are some examples: they zap brains with electricity during surgeries (with patients' permission, of course), they use implanted electrodes to record electrical activity produced by neurons, or they place experienced meditators in magnetic resonance imaging scanners. Such studies show, for example, that if you stimulate parts of the default network of someone's brain — so the regions of the cortex that activate when you think about the past or envision the future — you may cause that person to daydream and spontaneously recall memories. And if you run one-millisecond electrical pulses through the almond-shaped amygdala, you can cause déjà vécu—kind of like déjà vu on steroids—an illusion of having lived a whole sequence of events already, one that is longer, less fleeting, and less easy to dismiss than déjà vu. The amygdala, the region that is very likely involved in thinking, is also one of the main brain structures that can help explain how our minds and bodies are interconnected. The keyword here is fear.

Ghosts and Hormones

It was about ten o'clock at night when SM, a thirty-year-old woman, was on her way home. The area was deserted, with only the sounds of choir music floating out of a nearby church interrupting the stillness. As SM walked past a small park, she noticed a man sitting on a bench. She thought he looked "drugged-out," but when he motioned her to come over, she obliged. The moment SM approached the man, he jumped up, pulled her by the shirt, and pressed a knife to her throat, shouting, "I'm going to cut you, bitch!"

If I had been in SM's place, I would have been shaking with panic. My heart would have raced and my palms would have been drenched with sweat. Yet SM felt no fear. She replied calmly, "If you're going to kill me, you're gonna have to go through my God's angels first." Then, slowly, she walked away, leaving the stunned man behind. The very next night she strolled home through the same park. No anxiety, no panic, nothing.

SM, as she is known to medical researchers, suffers from Urbach-Wiethe disease, a rare genetic disorder that has left her with a damaged amygdala. Since this brain region acts as a quick detector of potential threats, SM is basically fearless. She picks up dangerous snakes with her bare hands and watches horror movies without flinching. Even one of the world's scariest haunted houses, the Waverly Hills Sanatorium in Louisville, Kentucky, wasn't enough to unsettle her. For one experiment, scientists took SM on a tour of the Waverly Hills Sanatorium hoping to observe her reactions to the local "demons"—Sanatorium's workers dressed to look scary. What they saw was pure spunk: SM never hesitated to walk around murky corners and laughed at the "demons," even trying to chat them up. Other people, meanwhile, lagged behind her and screamed in fright whenever "monsters" and "ghosts" startled them.

SM's boldness may seem enviable, but unfortunately it has dangerous consequences. SM has fallen victim to numerous crimes, from domestic violence to death threats and assaults. Without fear, she makes mistakes other people tend to avoid—like approaching a drugged-out-looking guy in a dark, empty park. Her fight-or-flight response just doesn't activate properly.

If you are like me and most amygdala-lesion-free people, you would likely feel anxious in a deserted public space at nighttime. Faced with a criminal and a knife, you would probably experience a certain mixture of emotions (fear, panic, anger), sharper attention, and physical sensations such as a racing heart, sweaty palms, and difficulty swallowing. That's a fight-or-flight response, your mind and body interacting to save your life, just as it worked for our ancestors on the savanna.

The fight-or-flight response evolved to aid us in either wrestling dangerous animals and humans or making a successful escape. The rate and force of heart contractions increase. Blood pressure goes up. More blood is pumped into your skeletal muscles to help you move more quickly, boosting your strength. Your bronchial tubes dilate, which makes breathing easier. The pupils in your eyes dilate as well, so you can focus your sight better. In extreme situations some people may even empty their bladders or bowels—that's also an evolved part of the fight-or-flight response. After all, if you have no extra weight in your abdomen, you can flee faster.

Even though these days lions are uncommon on the streets of Manhattan or London, the fight-or-flight response, known also as the "stress response," is something most of us know well. Your boss says he "needs to talk"? Fear, racing heart. Someone flips you off in traffic? Anger, sweaty palms. Exams are starting? Anxiety, stomach issues (bowels emptying to facilitate fleeing). It all creates a cascade of emotions and physical changes which, if chronic, can result in heart disease, premature aging, and even particularly bad colds. There are four main pathways connecting your mind and your body, all of them related to the stress response: the sympathomedullary axis, the HPA axis, the immune system, and about three pounds of microbes that are living in your gut.

When you are faced with a lion or with an angry boss, the first changes in your body happen in split seconds. That's your sympathomedullary pathway activating. It's a very primitive system that works whether you want it to or not. The amygdala, the fear centre, sends a message down to your adrenal glands, two grape-sized organs that sit on top of your kidneys. The adrenal glands then release a soup of hormones which includes the famed adrenaline. Your blood is diverted away from your gut and kidneys—admittedly rather useless systems in a fight—to those parts of your body that are more vital for saving your life, such as the skeletal muscles and the brain. You feel pumped up.

You are almost ready to go, but your body is not yet done. A second system kicks in, a more complicated one known as the hypo-thalamus-pituitary-adrenal axis. Once alarmed by the amygdala, a part of the brain called the hypothalamus starts a hormonal cascade that again ends up revving up the adrenal glands, just a different part of them. Another cocktail spills into the bloodstream, this one containing hormones such as cortisol.

If you've heard about stress, you've probably heard about corti-sol. This hormone has a bad reputation as the evil-incarnate side-kick of stress, to the point that *Psychology Today* once called it "public health enemy number one." On the purely physiological side, cor-tisol has been linked to weight gain, diabetes, cancer, and heart disease. On the psychological side, it's been shown to spur aggres-sion and antisocial behaviours. Although now it seems clear that cortisol connects the body and the mind in multiple ways, when it was first discovered in the 1940s, it was touted as a miracle cure for stress and rheumatoid arthritis. The knowledge that it has much more complex effects on the body and the psyche came only later. And it all started with a twenty-nine-year-old woman from Kokomo, Indiana.

Bad Stress, Good Stress

During World War Two, rumours abounded that the Nazis were developing a miracle cure for stress so that their pilots could zoom around in their Messerschmitts with no regard to speed and alti-tude. The Germans were, supposedly, importing tons of bovine adrenal glands from Argentina and extracting some "mysterious humour" out of them. By then it was known to science that cows without adrenal glands died when subjected to even minimal stress, so the argument that the extract would make pilots stress-resistant seemed plausible. With hopes for outstanding military gains, the American government invested tons of money into the research on the mysterious humour, giving it the third priority after penicillin and antimalarials.

The cash injections into research on adrenal glands provided a great boost to the work of three scientists, Americans Phillip Hench and Edward Kendall and their Polish colleague Tadeusz Reichstein. With a steady supply of nine hundred pounds a week of adrenal glands from some unlucky cows, the three researchers perfected the production of something they named "compound E," which we now call cortisol. But before anyone managed to turn "compound E" into a courage pill, the war ended.

With less need for pilot superpowers, the scientists went on to experiment with cortisol as a potential cure for rheumatoid arthritis. In 1948 they recruited a Mrs. Gardner from Indiana for experimental treatments. Young Mrs. Gardner's arthritis was so bad that on most days the pain wouldn't allow her to walk or even get out of bed. On September 21, 1948, Mrs. Gardner received initial injections of large doses of cortisol. At first, nothing seemed to happen, but after four days of treatment, her pain was completely gone. When the scientists visited her room in Saint Mary's Hospital in Rochester, Minnesota, they found her exercising, lifting her hands up over her head—a feat she had been previously incapable of. On September 28, Mrs. Gardner left the hospital and went on a shopping spree in downtown Rochester. She appeared completely cured.

Then, after about two weeks, the problems began. But it wasn't pain that was troubling Mrs. Gardner this time, it was her mood. It would swing from depressed to euphoric and then back. Occasionally, she would become psychotic, and ended up admitted to Saint Mary's locked psychiatric ward. Once her cortisol injections were stopped, the troubles with her mind cleared up. She refused to take cortisol ever again, choosing pain over psychosis.

For their discovery of cortisol, Hench, Kendall, and Reichstein received the Nobel Prize in 1950, but it took many more decades for researchers to get a better understanding of its role in our stress response and mind-brain connections. Modern science shows that cortisol is just one cog in the machinery of stress, the HPA axis, which involves a whole cascade of hormones. First, there is the corticotrophin-releasing hormone secreted by the brain's hypothalamus into the blood. The hormone triggers a pea-sized organ at the base of your brain, the pituitary gland, to pump out adrenocorticotropic hormone, which then flows all the way down to the kidneys, where it switches on the production of hormones such as aldosterone and cortisol from the adrenal glands.

Your body is readying for the fight or flight—and its consequences. Since you need energy to both flee and battle, cortisol will provide you with a fuel boost by breaking down proteins and fat from long-lasting sources, such as your muscles, to raise blood glucose levels. Both cortisol and aldosterone will also raise your blood pressure by constricting your blood vessels (cortisol) and increasing salt and water retention (aldosterone). Lions and angry bosses beware—you are ready to fight.

If you are lucky and the lion turns around and strides away into the sunset, your stress axis will calm down, and all systems will go back to baseline. The hypothalamus will detect the raised levels of cortisol in the blood and put a halt to its production within forty to sixty minutes after the anxiety-inducing event. Meanwhile, a cousin branch of your sympathomedullary pathway will activate a rest-and-digest response, which calms down all the previous changes in your adrenaline-releasing system. You begin to relax.

Here is a problem, though. On an African savanna, the things that caused our ancestors anxiety or anger usually happened fast and resolved fast (the lion went away: problem gone); the things that today arouse our negative emotions are, by contrast, often low-intensity but long-lasting. Mortgage stress activates the HPA axis as surely as carnivorous cats do, yet mortgages tend to stick around longer than predators. Same for traffic, work issues, loneliness, over-scheduling, worrying about your kids' college admissions, and so on.

Unfortunately, when activation of the HPA axis becomes chronic, troubles start to mount. The axis becomes dysregulated and the levels of cortisol stay constantly up. The hypothalamus begins to shrink (yes, you've heard it right—stress shrinks your brain, or at least some parts of it). What may grow, though, is your stomach. Since cortisol takes up fat from places such as the legs and arms, and then lets it settle around the waist, you may grow chunkier in your mid-section—that's why some researchers use a high waist-to-hip ratio as a marker for chronic stress. The interplay between fat and cortisol may also lead to insulin resistance, and then to diabetes, cardiovascular disease, and even cancer.

By modifying cortisol levels and the activation of the sympatho-medullary pathway, your psyche can change your body all the way down to your DNA, changing the expression of your genes. Like a finger on a light switch, stress hormones turn genes on and off. This includes genes related to the immune system. If a person is under chronic stress, the stress pathways flip on genes involved in inflammation, and switch off those responsible for the antiviral response. From the savanna perspective, it made sense. Back then chronic stress usually meant being outside the camp—away from viruses usually carried by fellow tribe members—and at a higher risk of wounds, which can get infected by bacteria. Our chronically stressed ancestors got scratched by thorny branches while chasing prey, mauled by predators, or slashed by enemies. The immune system, like everything in nature, takes energy to run and compromises had to be made. So down went antiviral protection, and up went inflammation, which is great for fighting bacteria in an oozing wound.

Today, however, this conserved response to adversity is far from helpful. What it means in practice is that persistent worries over jobs, kids, and mortgages make us less resistant to viruses, from the common cold to the flu, and more prone to inflammation, which in the long run leads to diabetes, stroke, heart disease, and cancer. Out of the ten leading causes of death, chronic inflammation contributes to at least seven.

Intertwined with the stress pathways, the immune system is itself a great connector between our minds and bodies, helping explain how our emotions and thoughts affect our health. This is a hot new area of research, recently christened "immunopsychiatry." Your immune system is directly wired to your brain via nerves and neurotransmitters. Think of the last time you were sick with a virus. How did you feel, psychologically? Probably gloomy and miserable, wishing to stay bundled up in bed all day. People often assume that such lethargy is a direct result of the virus messing with their bodies, but that's not really the case. That unpleasant feeling is mostly in your head—you'd quite likely be fine going out to party. This so-called "sickness behaviour" is actually caused by your own immune system, or your pro-inflammatory cytokines, to be precise. Cytokines are proteins that regulate the inflammatory response, helping fight various pathogens and heal wounds. But they also induce the behavioural and psychological changes that tie us to the bed when ill.

Sickness behaviour likely evolved so that ailing people would not spread the infection to the other members of the tribe, and so that they would not fall easy victim in spats with healthy others. That's why when you are under the weather you feel like hiding away and you may tolerate only a handful of your most trusted people.

While "lying miserably in bed" and "no energy" may be a good description of someone with a flu, it may also be a fitting description of someone with depression. Science is beginning to uncover the surprising links between depression, stress, and inflammation. When your body spews pro-inflammatory cytokines in particularly large quantities or for long periods of time, you are at a higher risk of becoming depressed.

One meta-analysis showed that about a quarter of patients with hepatitis C who are treated with the cytokine interferon-alpha develop depression as a side effect. In animals, injections with both infectious bacteria and pro-inflammatory cytokines cause depression, too. Who will succumb to the immune system–induced gloom likely depends on their stress resilience and coping style. Studies on mice and rats show that only those who are susceptible to stress and deal with challenges passively, instead of grabbing their rodent lives by the horns, end up with elevated levels of pro-inflammatory cytokines, depression and, as a consequence, heart disease. In humans, too, depression is associated with early mortality. When this is not the result of suicide, it is often caused by cardiovascular problems, with inflammation the likely culprit.

The links between the psyche, depression, and inflammation are complicated and bidirectional. Chronic stress can raise levels of pro-inflammatory cytokines and result in depression. Yet inflammation per se can make you feel desolate, too. For this reason anti-inflammatory drugs are now being proposed as treatment for depression in patients who don't respond to traditional remedies. Should you then take ibuprofen whenever you feel a touch of blues? Research has not addressed this question yet, but my guess would be: probably not, since in my opinion routine downing of pills is rarely a solution. But for those with major depression, anti-inflammatory drugs may offer real hope.

How, exactly, can tiny, inflammation-inducing proteins that circulate in your blood affect the thoughts and emotions in your brain? The answer isn't completely clear, but research reveals that they can both cross into the brain directly and also transmit the message to your central computer via a nerve called the vagus. The vagus, which is the longest nerve that emerges directly from the brain, seems crucial in the connections between the mind and the body. It may even be behind the ultimate mind-body events: psychogenic or "voodoo" deaths.

Deadly Hens, Drownings, and HRV Monitors

In 1682, Girolamo Merolla da Sorrento, an Italian missionary, travelled through the Congo and reported a story of a young African man who stayed at a friend's house. The host offered wild hen for breakfast—a food that was taboo in the young African's culture—yet lied about it, claiming the bird was something else. The young African ate happily and soon forgot about the whole thing. But years later the two met again and the cook asked if the young man would like to taste some wild hen. When faced with stern refusal—after all, the food was strictly banned by a local "wizard"—the cook informed the youth that he had broken the taboo already in the past. The young man began to tremble, completely overcome by fear. Within twenty-four hours, he was dead.

Meat consumption may be bad for your cholesterol levels and cardiovascular health in general, but by itself it can't make you collapse on the spot. The young Congolese likely fell victim to a psychogenic or "voodoo" death—a sudden, unexplained demise initiated by a belief in a mortal curse. Reports of psychogenic deaths abound across the planet, from the islands of the Pacific to South America, Africa, Australia, and New Zealand.

The clue to what may be causing psychogenic deaths comes from some cases of drownings. About 10 to 15 percent of people who die plunging into an ocean or a river have no water in their lungs, indicating that they haven't, in fact, drowned at all. In animal experiments similar cases have been attributed to the overstimulation of the vagus nerve. Such sudden vagal death, some scientists believe, could also explain the mortal power of voodoo curses.

The vagus nerve goes from the base of your skull down your neck and along your trachea to your heart and then wanders lower to your abdomen, where it innervates the gastrointestinal tract. It's responsible for your breathing, swallowing, and digestion. It's also responsible for the way your heart beats. The vagus is a major nerve of the autonomic nervous system and as such also plays a role in the fight-and-flight response. In a way, it's on the flip side of the sympathomedullary pathway and the HPA axis—it calms down the system after stress, bringing on relaxation once an adrenaline-pumping event is over. Your heart slows down, your breathing steadies, your digestion picks up again.

Sudden overstimulation of the vagus nerve can be a bad thing—it can basically shut you down, slowing your heart so much that it stops, causing a psychogenic death or a drowning-like event. Yet milder increases in vagal activity are quite good for you, keeping your body and mind relaxed and in top condition. Some research actually suggests that we could even treat chronic pain and depression by applying electrical stimulation to the vagus nerve. A common measure used by scientists that reflects the workings of the vagus nerve is heart rate variability. If you haven't come across it yet reading fitness and health magazines, you soon may. Heart rate variability, or HRV for short, is emerging as a particularly valuable indicator of the health of the vagus nerve, the proper functioning of our fight-and-flight response, the mind-body connection, and even potential longevity.

It may seem like a good thing to have a heart that beats as evenly as the most coordinated marching band, but it is not. In fact, the more varied your heart rate the better. In a normal heart, the time that lapses between two successive beats is always slightly different—even breathing in and out changes the rate. These tiny differences between heartbeats are what is measured as heart rate variability. If the variability is high, it means that your heart is capable of quick adjustments to the changing environment. It can mobilize resources fast and relax fast. In the evolutionary past, if you could control your fear, suppress unwanted thoughts, and mobilize your inner resources, you were certainly better off when faced with a large mouth full of sharp teeth that was trying to eat you. It meant that your vagus nerve, the link between your brain and your heart, was working well.

But when we are chronically stressed, our fight-and-flight response can get stuck in high gear and prevent the vagus from initiating the relaxation response. The system becomes dysregulated, with the HRV permanently low. Lack of resilience and proper emotional regulation, worrying a lot, anxiety, loneliness—these have all been linked to low HRV. Poor physical health may follow. More and more research is now showing that low HRV can lead to diabetes, cardiovascular disease, and even an earlier death.

The good news is that you can monitor your HRV at home and evaluate whether your health interventions are working. The easiest way is to buy a chest-strap heart monitor from a company like Wahoo or Polar and download a free app that will analyze the data. When I first turned on my newly acquired HRV monitor, I hoped for a readout indicating that I had a body of a twentysomething. The reality was less rosy. After precisely two minutes of sitting still, I discovered that I had a body of someone . . . exactly my age. Oh, well. Luckily for me studies show that lifestyle changes, such as yoga, can improve HRV quickly—the difference can be seen in as little as eight weeks (more on that in chapter 10).

Besides sending messages from your brain to your heart and back, the vagus nerve, which reaches deep into your body, also functions as an information highway between your central computer and your gut—or, to be more precise, between your central computer and the trillions of bacteria residing in your intestines. To learn more about how such tiny creatures can connect minds and bodies, I went mouse-catching in Oxfordshire, UK.

Of Mice and Guts

At 7:30 a.m. one sunny June morning, I crossed through a timber gate into Wytham Great Wood, a forested area just seven miles away from the University of Oxford. After a half-hour walk alone through a dark forest, during which I grew increasingly anxious, I finally reached a Swiss-style chalet, which, had I not known better, I would have taken for abandoned. The place was overgrown with weeds and surrounded by piles of discarded animal cages. Gingerly I stepped inside. There, in a tiny room that smelled of disinfectant, Aura Raulo was sweeping mouse poop out of a metal container. Noticing me, the young researcher smiled and took off her latex gloves to shake my hand.

I had contacted Raulo a few weeks before to talk about her research on how sociality influences the gut microbiome, and vice versa. That's when she suggested I join her and her team in Wytham Great Wood, where they catch wild British wood mice, run behavioural tests on them, and analyze their poop.

Very early in the morning of my arrival, rectangular, metal traps were set in the forest surrounding the chalet. Each carefully numbered trap contained something few mice can resist: peanuts. "Some of them like peanuts so much, they can be caught in the traps again and again," Raulo told me. As she showed me around, stepping carefully over thorny shrubs and nettles, she pointed to little yellow flags marking barely visible holes in the undergrowth: mouse burrows. Beside the burrows, wireless loggers equipped with motion sensors were ready to turn on whenever something warm moved past them. The equipment would also read the tiny tags that each mouse carried. "This way we can see who goes in and out," Raulo told me, then added with a laugh, "I think these are the most intensely monitored mice in the UK."

Back at the chalet's cramped lab, Raulo opened the trap to release mouse number 931 into her gloved hand. She measured and weighed him, took a fur sample to check cortisol levels, and collected the poop that he had conveniently left on the cotton wool bedding inside the container—it would be analyzed for microbial content later on. After that, mouse number 931 was sent off to a "personality assay chamber" in the next room.

The mouse was placed in the middle of an empty cage and left alone, his movements tracked by a hidden camera. He spent the next five minutes wandering shyly around, sniffing at corners. You can tell a lot about a mouse's personality by the way it behaves when placed in a new environment, Raulo told me. The brave, outgoing ones will calmly check everything out. The anxious ones will end up running in circles. And some will be so terrified they will just freeze in one spot. If you compare this behavioural data with information gathered from the poop on the gut microbiome, and if you do this over and over, you can get some idea of the links between bacteria that reside in the intestines and the rodent personality.

What Raulo does as well—and what is her prime focus—is to investigate how social networks influence the gut microbiome. She analyzes the data from the logging devices outside the burrows, checking who hangs out with whom, and then runs it by the poop microbiome stats. She has already discovered that not only do mice share bacteria with their friends, but also that the more diverse friendships they have, the more diverse their microbiomes—which is generally an indicator of a healthy gut.

She believes a similar pattern may apply to humans, too. "Imagine you have just two friends. One of them is a famous disco queen and the other is a famous metal singer. Because they represent very distinct social networks they have very different microbiomes. If you are the link between the two of them you get the richness of all their bacteria combined. A similar thing would happen if you were from a multicultural family, with relatives in different countries," Raulo said. Some early research on humans does confirm that we may transfer friendly bacteria between ourselves the way Raulo's mice do. One such study showed, for example, that roller derby players exchange microbes with opposing teams during tournaments. Family members, meanwhile, share bacteria with each other and even their dogs.

Other experiments suggest that changes in the gut microbiome can influence personality. If you breed mice devoid of any beneficial gut bacteria, the rodents will be loners, preferring to sit away from all the others. And if you recolonize their intestines with microbes, their personality will change once again—back to social. So how do you breed germ-free mice? You make sure they are born by Caesarean section so that they don't get any beneficial microbes from their mothers, have them live in sterile quarters, and feed them purified water and food. If that reminds you of people you may know, that's bad news. Germ-free rodents have been shown to have overreactive HPA axes and to be less resilient to stress.

Again, human studies point in a similar direction. In the Philippines, for instance, young people in their twenties who had a lot of contact with animal feces in infancy have been proven to be more resistant to stress as adults. In case "contact with animal feces" does not sound particularly appealing to you as a mood-boosting intervention, the good news is that probiotics work, too. When a group of American volunteers drank probiotic-rich fermented milk for about a month, their brain activity patterns changed—suggesting that their processing of emotions had changed—in a way that could make them, for example, less prone to overreact to fear- or anxiety-inducing situations. A similar experiment showed that consumption of the bacteria *Bifidobacterium longum*, which you can find in kefir or miso soup, reduces cortisol release and dampens stress.

And in case miso soup doesn't do the trick, there are always fecal transfers (back to poop, sorry). In one particularly revealing study scientists have taken stool from depressed patients and transplanted it into some unlucky rats. The rodents became instantly depressed themselves, losing interest in things they used to enjoy. Fecal transfers have even more striking results if done within the same species. Take poop from an anxious mouse and insert it into a second mouse, and your mouse number two will become anxious as well. Same thing happens with poop from inquisitive rodents—it can turn others inquisitive and curious, too. Which made me wonder: does having gloomy friends turn you gloomy, too, since you trade microbes through hugs and skin contact? Should I avoid touching people with particularly dark or unpleasant temperaments? Sounds a bit extreme, but maybe better safe than sorry? Dear scientists, please research.

Just the way the bacteria in your intestines can influence your mood, on the flip side, worry and anxiety can damage your gut microbiome, too. When experimental animals are stressed, the composition of germs in their poop changes in response—for the worse. Which means that every time I worry that my daughter's runny nose will develop into a full-blown sickness, or when I stress over a deadline, or panic that climate change will soon kill us all, I'm hurting the beneficial microbes in my intestines, while giving a boost to the harmful ones. The reason for this is that stress hormones tamper with the physiology of the gut, modifying the habitat for the bacteria in a way that's unfriendly to the good guys.

So how exactly can brain talk with the gut? One such communication channel is the vagus nerve; another is neurotransmitters such as serotonin and dopamine. Besides being produced by the brain, neurotransmitters can also be synthesized by the intestinal microbiota. If you lived in a completely sterile environment and had no gut bacteria whatsoever, like the germ-free lab rats, the serotonin system in your brain wouldn't develop properly, playing havoc with your emotions. Gut bacteria can also work on your brain through the metabolites they produce, such as short-chain fatty acids. Butyrate, a short-chain fatty acid that's a cousin chemical to the obnoxious butyric acid (responsible for the sour-bitter stench of rancid butter), may help the growth of new neurons in the brain and survival of the old ones. What's more, intestinal microbes can also tweak your immune system and regulate your HPA axis.

Besides chatting with your central nervous system and having an influence on our moods and behaviours, friendly gut bacteria are essential for our physical health, too. Messed-up intestinal microflora have been implicated in many diseases, including diabetes, multiple sclerosis, rheumatoid arthritis, and allergies. On the flip side, transplants of poop from young donors can prolong life—at least in fish.

When researchers from the Max Planck Institute for Biology of Ageing in Germany made middle-aged turquoise killifish nibble on the feces of their younger companions, the animals lived 37 percent longer than those that were not provided with such unusual food. From a human perspective, that would be like extending the current American average lifespan of 78 years to 107. Imagine that. Fecal transplants are already used to treat diabetes and obesity in people—although for now, no one seems to be testing this therapy for human longevity.

Of course it's far too early to recommend poop supplements from youthful donors to people who want to live long—assuming anyone would be up for trying these (I know I wouldn't). And maybe we won't have to. Maybe just thinking you are getting a miracle treatment can suffice. When it comes to mind-body connections, the placebo effect can truly work wonders.

Water Injections and Sham Surgery

Mr. Wright had cancer. An untreatable one that had spread all through his body. He couldn't even breathe without extra oxygen. He really wanted to live, though, and asked his physician to administer him a new experimental drug called Krebiozen. But the doctor knew Krebiozen was worthless, so without Mr. Wright's knowledge, gave him water injections instead, curious to see what would happen. To the physician's surprise, the sick man improved dramatically. Within days, Mr. Wright was basically symptom-free—he was so well, in fact, that once he was discharged from the hospital, he flew himself home in his own airplane. His good health lasted until one day, two months later, the American Medical Association published a statement saying that Krebiozen did nothing for treating cancer. Once Mr. Wright got the depressing news, his health plummeted. He got readmitted to a hospital, and two days later, he was dead.

The use of placebos in medicine is probably as old as humanity itself. In ancient Egypt, the sick were treated with concoctions made from crocodile dung and swine teeth. In medieval Europe, you might have received such cures as ground-up "unicorn's horn," which was in fact just ivory, or something that was supposedly a "crystallized tear from the eye of a deer bitten by a snake" (usually a gallstone). These days, even though most of us would not fall for unicorn pills, many people happily spring for homeopathic drugs, which are placebos, too.

Which does not mean these things don't work—research shows that placebos are actually quite effective. They help for conditions as varied as Parkinson's disease, depression, chronic pain, and nausea. Even a sham arthroscopic knee surgery works as well as a real one. What's more, placebos work even if you know you are getting nothing but a sugar pill. In one study of cancer survivors suffering from fatigue, taking a placebo that was clearly marked as being just that helped ease the symptoms as much as a standard treatment.

One reason placebos work is because of expectations (even if you know it's a placebo). In a way, when faced with a sugar pill that promises to help us feel better we act like the famed Pavlov's dogs, which would salivate at a mere sound of a bell. When we see a doctor in a white coat with a well-equipped medical office, and we smell the scent of hospital-grade disinfectant, our central nervous system recalls when similar things happened to us in the past and helped us get healthy, conditioning us to improve this time, too. That's why the more medicalized the placebo, the better it works. A pill given by a doctor works better than a pill given by a friend. A drug administered in a hospital works better than one given at home. A fake injection works better than a pill—simply because it's more invasive, which makes it appear more serious and real.

Yet, as renowned placebo researcher Fabrizio Benedetti told me, there is no single explanation for why placebos work because there isn't a single placebo effect. "These are complex phenomena that involve many mechanisms," he said. They may act through neurotransmitters such as endocannabinoids and dopamine or through the HPA axis. When scientists put people who have received placebos into functional magnetic resonance imaging scanners, they can see the effects of the sham treatments in the activation patterns of the brain, for instance in the amygdala.

One mechanism particularly stands out when it comes to placebos—I'm talking about the opioid system. Opioids are substances akin to heroin and morphine that are churned out by your own body so that you can deal with pain. Opioids are the reason you may not perceive pain when under huge stress, which makes sense from an evolutionary perspective: it was better for our ancestors not to fixate on unpleasant yet distracting sensations coming from, say, a mauled limb, while fighting wild animals. Today, when you take a placebo that's supposed to ease your aches, you start to stimulate production of these natural painkillers. Your mind and your body act together to help you improve.

⧗

Our feelings, thoughts, and social behaviours can influence our health and longevity. It's no magic. The connection between the mind and the body is a very ancient one and is based on the mechanisms that helped our ancestors fight or flee for their lives when faced with a threat. Your HPA axis, the sympathomedullary pathway, the vagus nerve, the immune system, the trillions of microbes in the gut—they all respond to the messages coming from your brain to keep you alive. Your emotions, from fear to anger to happiness, help inform these systems about the state of your body and the environment, preparing them for action. If the stress response is initiated, a cascade of hormones washes through your body, changing the way your muscles, heart, lungs, and digestive system work. Once the threat is gone, the relaxation response kicks in. The vagus nerve does its job. You feel calm, composed.

These days, however, that ancient stress response often malfunctions. We may be lonely, switching on the inflammatory response of someone stranded away from the tribe. We live fast, under constant mental pressure, bombarded by challenges. The HPA axis becomes dysregulated, and the vagus nerve has no chance of starting the relaxation response. The stress systems stay turned on, damaging different organs in the process, so we end up with permanently raised blood pressure, clogged arteries, or insulin resistance. With time, that can lead to diabetes, heart disease, or a shortened lifespan.

You can monitor your heart rate variability for the condition of your vagus nerve. You can check your blood for signs of chronic inflammation. You can even get your gut microbiota tested for its health. The practical tips about such services can be found on this book's website. But you probably know in your gut (the proverbial one) whether your stress and relaxation response might be out of whack. Luckily science has revealed many different approaches and techniques that we can use to improve the mind-body connection, from the functioning of the HPA axis to the quality of the gut microbiota. Drinking kefir and eating miso soup certainly won't hurt, but changing your mindset and the way you live in society is even more important: improving close relationships (which, according to studies, may lower mortality by about 45 percent), working on empathy and kindness (44 percent), adding mindfulness and volunteering (22 percent).

All these work to boost health and longevity through mechanisms mentioned in this chapter. But there is more. Just as we've evolved the stress response to deal with imminent threats, we've also evolved to be social creatures, relying on one another for help. That's why a cocktail of so-called social hormones, such as oxytocin, serotonin, and vasopressin, also play a vital role in both our mental and physical well-being, connecting the mind and the body. It can explain, for instance, why holding hands and looking others in the eye can be good for your health.

A FEW SUGGESTIONS TO BOOST YOUR LONGEVITY

Take good care of your HPA axis so it doesn't become chronically activated—traffic squabbles are not lions trying to eat you. Have your doctor check out your heart rate variability (HRV) or buy a devise to measure it at home. It'll give you an idea of how your vagus nerve and relaxation response are working. If you are depressed and standard pills don't seem to do the trick, ask your doctor for anti-inflammatory drugs—our immune systems and brains are intricately connected. Tend to the microbes in your gut: don't overdo antibiotics or antibacterial cleaning products; eat lots of fermented foods such as miso or kefir; spend time getting dirty in nature. Keep diverse friendships. Give lot of hugs to your cheerful, easygoing friends and, through microbial exchange, their attitude may rub off on you, too. Profit from the placebo effect—it may work even if you know the treatment is a sham.

3

A SNIFF OF LOVE

*How Social Hormones Influence
Our Relationships and Longevity*

IN MY HAND, the blue-white bottle of OxyLuv felt just like any other nasal spray—a decongestant, perhaps, something I might use to relieve the symptoms of a bad cold. Yet this day I wasn't treating a stuffy nose. Instead, I was targeting potential deficiencies in my social skills.

I removed the cap from the bottle, tilted my head forward, and slid the cold, white nozzle into my left nostril. I sprayed, inhaled, and then repeated the process on the other side. Then it was show-time. Within a few minutes I was either going to feel overwhelming love toward the entire human population of earth, or, alternatively, get a nosebleed.

According to the producer's website, OxyLuv is supposed to "create feelings of trust between others" and reduce my "social fears, anxiety, stress." Each spray delivered to my brain ten international units of oxytocin, dubbed by the media as the "love" or "cuddle" hormone, and which, as a hefty pile of scientific studies shows, makes people more social and friendly, improving relationships.

Fifteen minutes after my first OxyLuv shot, I began to feel more serene, as if someone had wrapped me in a blanket of calm. I looked at my husband, who was sitting across the table, and smiled. All was fine in the world. With the extra dose of oxytocin reaching my amygdala and the anterior cingulate cortex, I should be more empathic today. Maybe I would be kinder to my husband, boosting marital love. Maybe I would make new friends, or bond better with the old ones. As a result, I should prolong my life.

Oxytocin is a protein-like molecule that neurons use to communicate with each other. Outside of the brain, it can also act as a hormone, regulating many different processes in the body. Oxytocin evolved about 700 million years ago, long before the first animals set their paws on land. Over the millennia, oxytocin and its close relatives became widespread in the animal kingdom, helping with reproduction and sociality. They induce milk letdown in lactating mammals, be it squirrels or humans. They cause contractions of the gut in worms and contractions of the uterus during human childbirth. They help leeches twist. They incite male cichlid fish to be better fathers. And when you see a dog looking faithfully into his master's eyes, oxytocin is at work, too.

These are not just some spurious connections. There are very good biological reasons why oxytocin, together with other hormones such as vasopressin, endorphins, dopamine, and serotonin, play a vital role both in our social lives and in our health, tying them together. These so-called social neuropeptides are the reason why being neighbourly or having a happy marriage may add years to your lifespan. Neurochemical links between sociality and physiology are crucial for our species. Some researchers even argue that social hormones have actually made us human. According to one theory called "the neurochemical hypothesis for the origin of hominids" (yes, it's a mouthful), selection for high amounts of dopamine and serotonin in our brains tilted our personalities toward less aggression and higher levels of cooperation. And while over our evolutionary history we've become kinder, calmer, and friendlier, at the same time the scleras of our eyes turned white, our lips became pinker, and our brains shrank.

What Makes a Good Pet

On one YouTube video, Boris and Sophie, two cute pets, show off their tricks: they sit and lie down when prompted, then shake paws and spin in exchange for treats. If it weren't for their magnificent, bushy tails and unusually high-pitched yelps, the animals could be mistaken for dogs. In reality, Boris and Sophie are foxes—domesticated silver foxes from Siberia, to be precise.

In 1959 a Russian geneticist named Dmitry Belyaev set up an experiment to test a new research idea: he started breeding wild silver foxes, selecting the animals for their lack of aggression or fear toward humans. After a few years—or about eight to ten fox generations—a weird thing happened: some of the foxes started to resemble dogs in both their behaviour and looks. Today, the project continues even after Belyaev's death, and most of the domesticated silver foxes at the Siberian lab are tame creatures that are not only super-friendly, but also look considerably different from their wild ancestors.

They have floppy ears, short muzzles, and, often, white spots on the foreheads. But here is the thing: their looks are an unexpected side effect. Belyaev did not select the foxes for the floppiness of their ears or their forehead spots, no matter how cute. He selected them solely for their temperament. Yet what occurred was a whole set of appearance changes—something that scientists came to call the domestication syndrome. If you look at other species of domesticated animals, such as dogs, horses, donkeys, and rabbits, you may notice that they tend to have floppy ears, short snouts, small jaws, star-shaped marks on their foreheads, and smaller brains than their wild ancestors. Which brings us back to humans.

Richard Wrangham, a primatologist at Harvard University, believes that our ancestors self-domesticated themselves in recent evolutionary history, which resulted in milder tempers and more pro-social behaviours on one hand, and in smaller brains, smaller jaws, pink lips, white eye scleras, and flatter faces on the other (no floppy ears in our case—although I do wonder how that might have looked). And yes, you read that correctly: smaller brains. It is true that for the large part of our evolution our brains grew, but since late Pleistocene times, approximately thirty thousand years ago, they've actually slightly shrunk by about 10 percent. It might have been a side effect of selection for less reactive aggression, or in lay terms, better tempers.

Scientists believe that what may be responsible for such side effects, be it smaller brains or white forehead patches, is the neural crest. The neural crest is a group of stem cells found in the embryos of vertebrate animals—mammals, birds, fish, and so on—which, as the embryos develop, migrate throughout the body to give rise to different types of cells and tissues, including bones, cartilage, and melanocytes—a type of pigment-producing cell. At the same time, the neural crest cells also affect the levels of neuropeptides. In our evolutionary past, selection for better tempers meant selection for higher levels of oxytocin and serotonin, which in turn affected the neural crest cells and how far they could travel within the body. For example, when the neural crest cells don't make it to the top of the head of an animal, melanocytes won't develop there, resulting in depigmentation—hence the white forehead patches and white tail tips of domesticated animals. And that's also why humans have pink lips, and so do bonobo apes.

At first glance, bonobos may look very much like chimpanzees. That's hardly surprising, considering how closely the two species are related—they both belong to the genus *Pan*, which also makes them our nearest cousins. Yet, as zookeepers may tell you, there are some vital differences between these apes. While you might wander into a cage full of bonobos and leave unscathed, venturing into chimp territory is far more dangerous. Bonobos are nice and friendly, while the tempers of chimpanzees should not be taken lightly. Chimps kill one another, commit infanticide, and even attack their own mothers. Bonobos don't do that. No one has ever seen a bonobo murder another bonobo.

Wrangham suspects that bonobos, just like humans, have self-domesticated. That is also why, on closer inspection, they do look a bit different from chimps—they have the smaller jaws, more feminine-looking skulls (rounder, with less pronounced brow ridges), white palms, and pink lips of domesticated animals. And, in their brains they have twice as much serotonin, one of the social neuropeptides—an increase that has also been observed in the brains of tame Siberian foxes.

When humans, just like bonobos, self-domesticated, there were obviously no Russian geneticists to select us for friendliness—we did it all ourselves. In the case of bonobos, the richer and more predictable surroundings in which they lived as compared to chimps allowed females to reject overly aggressive males. Yet in the case of our ancestors, Wrangham argues, it wasn't mobilization of females but rather language that helped us self-select for tolerance and mild tempers.

And if you feel like pointing out that humans, with our genocides and wars, don't appear particularly bunny-like or docile, Wrangham has an answer to that, too. It all boils down to a difference between proactive and reactive aggression. Reactive aggression is the type common among chimps—someone makes you angry, so you bite their head off, sometimes literally. Proactive aggression, on the other hand, the premeditated scheming that can lead to dropping nuclear bombs on other members of your own species, is governed by very different neural pathways in the brain.

Our evolutionary selection likely went like this: imagine you had an aggressive and untrustworthy bully in your tribe. Other males would gather, and talk up a plan to get rid of the guy. They would choose the time and place—"By the old baobab? At noon?"—and, well, get rid of the guy, maybe with the help of a spear or two. Among some tribes, such capital punishment is actually quite common. Papua New Guinea's Etoro people, for instance, eliminate about 9 percent of men this way, inadvertently purging their ranks of the bullies' genes for low oxytocin and serotonin.

Over our evolutionary history, selecting for more friendly hominins meant selecting those with higher levels of social hormones circulating in their bodies. After our line split from Neanderthals, such a push for more oxytocin, paired with neural crest–related depigmentation, likely changed the appearance of our eyes, too, making them quite unusual in the animal kingdom. Think of a typical wild mammal, say a deer or a zebra. Their eyes are all dark, like small lumps of coal. Human eyes, with white around the irises, certainly stand out. Of the dozens of primate species examined, only we have white scleras. That is also why, back in 2015, the photo of Nadia the gorilla went viral on the internet. In contrast to most members of her species, Nadia has white scleras, giving her a very human look.

The thing about white scleras is that without them, it's really hard to read much from the gaze of animals—not too much in the way of emotions, or even what the creature is looking at. Evolution of white scleras, prompted by self-domestication, helped our sociality even further. We could now communicate with others simply by looking into their eyes.

Today, our self-domesticated bodies and social minds are all interconnected. Oxytocin, serotonin, vasopressin, and other social hormones still play a vital role in linking our health and our behaviours. Yet scientists have a problem. It's not easy to study what's going on in our brains as we interact with each other (can't exactly cut them open). Luckily, however, there is one tiny animal species researchers can analyze instead, which offers us a unique window into the functions of several neuropeptides in both pro-social behaviours and health. I'm talking about prairie voles.

As rodents go, prairie voles are certainly among the cutest. Resembling a cross between a hamster and a mouse, they are round and fluffy, with black beady eyes and small, shapely ears. They may not look much like humans, but in many ways, they are actually rather similar to us. And it's not just their unusual penchant for alcohol (unlike most animals, prairie voles will choose booze over water). It's their monogamy, sociality, and parenting styles—all linked to the way their brains are wired for oxytocin.

Although prairie voles generally live in the grasslands of central North America, the most famous ones, at least from the perspective of neuroscience, inhabit the lab of Larry Young at Emory University in Atlanta. Here, though, the transparent plastic containers filled with wood shavings and occupied by prairie voles sit next to containers housing a species that in nature lives quite apart from prairie voles: montane voles of the North American mountains.

Young and his colleagues have been comparing the two cousin species for over two decades, and their work has greatly boosted our understanding of the role oxytocin plays in love, parenting, and friendships, both of the vole and of the human kind. Unlike the monogamous prairie voles, montane voles lead far more wild lifestyles—as far as sex goes, that is. While prairie voles form lifelong bonds, for montane voles it's all about casual rendezvous with as many partners as possible. And while prairie vole parents take care of their little ones together, with the fathers licking and grooming the kids just as the mothers do, montane vole dads prefer to leave childcare to the females.

Fascinated by the strikingly different approaches to family life between the two closely related species, researchers did what they tend to do in such situations: they opened up the brains of the animals to look for answers. Here's what they found: the monogamous voles have a very different pattern of oxytocin and vasopressin receptors in their brains as compared to their promiscuous cousins (receptors are something akin to on/off buttons that a neuropeptide can activate). In other words, their wiring for those hormones is completely different.

The more human-like prairie voles have the oxytocin receptors located in the part of the brain that is involved in addiction. If you block those receptors, the little rodents will not fall in lifelong love and won't care for their kids with the same devotion. On the other hand, manipulating genetics of montane voles so that their oxytocin receptors start to mimic those found in prairie voles makes them ditch their wanton ways and settle down in monogamy. And although playing with human genetics and then dissecting brains for research is a no-no in twenty-first-century science, certain inborn conditions also suggest that the way we are wired for oxytocin can affect our relationships with others.

Autism, Anti-Autism, and Oxytocin Genes

One of the first things Vanessa Coggshall noticed about her new-born daughter, Emmy, was her big smile. Even when the two were still at the hospital's maternity ward in Summit, New Jersey, Emmy would grin ear to ear in a fashion that's certainly not typical for little humans of just a few days of age. "I've never seen a baby with a smile like that," Coggshall says.

Now, at six years old, Emmy is a particularly cheerful and friendly kid. "She goes up to everybody and says, 'Hi my name is Emmy, what's your name?' She will often throw compliments at people. We might be in a grocery store and she would say to a woman there, 'I like your shirt. That's a nice colour on you,'" Coggshall says. As many parents of preschoolers, myself included, know well, kids that age are far more likely to hide shyly behind their parents' legs when faced by an adult stranger than to start small talk. Vanessa admits that Emmy's behaviour tends to throw people off. They often stare at her, surprised. But Emmy just shakes it off and moves on to the next person.

Sometimes called anti-autism, the condition that Emmy has is known as Williams syndrome. It's caused by a deletion of about twenty-seven genes which results in attraction to strangers, happy-go-lucky personality, and a penchant for looking everybody in the eye. It may all seem like a good thing, but there is a dark side to the condition, too: heart problems, decreased bone mineral density, diabetes, and, on the behavioural side—simply trusting others too much.

Williams syndrome is very rare—it affects only about one person in ten thousand. Yet it gives researchers a unique look into genetic influences on our social brains. People like Emmy tend to have particularly high levels of oxytocin and vasopressin in their blood, which is connected to the so-called pro-sociality gene, *GTF2I*—and the likely reason why they are so extraordinarily friendly and trusting.

Autism, too, scientists believe, may be connected to oxytocin wiring in the brain. Mice that don't have oxytocin receptor genes tend to behave in autistic ways—they have a penchant for repetitive behaviours, for instance. Also, some experiments have shown that spraying oxytocin into the noses of kids with autism may boost their social skills. But if you have someone with autism in your family, don't rush to stock up on OxyLuv just yet. The work on such treatments is still in the early stages.

People with Williams syndrome or autism may stand out when it comes to their oxytocin systems, but it's not as if the rest of us are equal where oxytocin genes and sociality are concerned. In fact, there exist many variations in oxytocin genes that can explain why not everyone has the same social temperament. You may be someone with the AA genotype, for example (not to be confused with type A personality). You can't say "Oh, I'm a type AA personality"—you may simply have the AA genotype of one oxytocin receptor gene.

Which, by the way, is not a particularly good thing. Research shows that people with an AA variant of an oxytocin receptor gene called *rs53576* are less empathic, have more trouble reading feelings from other people's faces, are judged as less friendly by others, and, if they are mothers, parent their kids with less sensitivity in times of parental conflict. People with the GG genotype, on the flip side, are generally more socially inclined and more attuned to the emotions of others. The GG genotype is the one you are more likely to have, since only 15 percent of people are type AA.

Scientists say that existence of these different genotypes makes sense from the evolutionary perspective. For our ancestors, safety was in numbers, so evolution favoured those who craved the bond with others, and hence may the GG genotype have survived. On the other hand, the group also needed people who were less upset by being alone, those who might venture far away and explore the environment, such as the carriers of the AA genotype.

Yet your oxytocin-related genes, no matter whether you are an AA type or GG type, are not the end of the story. They don't doom you to being more or less social nor do they determine how you will interact with others. Having the AA genotype doesn't mean you will certainly be a loner, and as a result, live less long. Your environment is important, too, whether it's your social network—or what gets sprayed up your nose.

The Elixir of Youth

On one late afternoon in 2007, several couples entered the unassuming steel-and-concrete buildings of the University of Zurich, and headed for the psychology lab—a scene that would repeat itself many times over the following six months. The men and women, in their twenties, thirties, and forties, were to take part in an experiment on the effects of oxytocin on relationships. First, everyone was asked to chew on a synthetic swab, something that looked like a third of a cigarette, which soaked up saliva. This way the levels of cortisol, the indicator of stress, could be measured. The couples were then given a list of potentially conflict-inducing topics (money, work, parenting, etc.) and asked to pick the two that they considered the most burning in their own relationship. Afterward, everyone was handed a nasal spray that resembled my OxyLuv, and told to puff five times in each nostril. Some people received oxytocin, and some unknowingly got placebo. When the drugs kicked in, it was time to fight. The couples were enclosed alone in a room with just a video camera recording and told to "discuss" the pre-chosen conflict issues. The squabbles began.

After the "conflict discussion," as the scientists euphemistically called it, saliva samples were taken repeatedly to measure the changing levels of cortisol. By dinnertime the experiment was over and the couples went home. For the researchers, though, the work was merely beginning. Months down the road, when all the behaviours recorded on video had been analyzed and the cortisol levels charted, the results were announced: the couples who took oxytocin not only had less cortisol in their saliva, they were also less nasty when fighting. Even though the oxytocin-drugged couples threw contemptuous remarks and rolled their eyes at each other just like everyone else did, they made up for such negative behaviours with more eye contact, smiles, and talking openly about feelings. That was crucial: a high ratio of positive to negative interactions is a great predictor of marital stability.

There are plenty of other studies that show that spraying oxytocin into the nose affects our social skills. It makes us better at reading facial expressions of emotions, such as telling whether someone is sad, tired, or just bored. It makes us more trusting. It can even make husbands stand further away from pretty women, as I've mentioned. When men in committed relationships were asked to find a spot at the "most comfortable" distance from a very attractive female experimenter, those who had previously received intranasal sprays of oxytocin opted for a distance of twenty-eight inches (71 cm). Those who only had the placebo preferred to stand considerably closer to the woman—twenty-two inches (56 cm) away, suggesting that without extra oxytocin, they behaved more like montane voles than the prairie ones, with faithfulness less on their minds.

Oxytocin not only makes us loyal, less quarrelsome, and more empathic, studies also show that it can directly affect our physical health, which would help explain the many links between sociality and longevity. The underlying reason here is this: nature is lazy. It reuses stuff. Just like your favourite mug may be for drinking coffee one day and then for storing pencils another, molecules such as oxytocin have been repeatedly repurposed for various functions over our evolutionary history. First, it was simply regulating water balance to prevent dehydration. Then it was immunity and metabolism. And then other functions were added, such as activating the milk letdown reflex during breastfeeding. From there nature repurposed oxytocin and related hormones for regulating our social behaviours. But it's all still connected. Changes to the system influence all the uses—just like changes to neural crest cells could both affect friendliness of foxes and create spots on their foreheads. If oxytocin levels surge in your body—say, because a scientist sprayed the neuropeptide into your nostrils—you may suddenly feel more lovey-dovey to the people around you, and your health may be affected, too.

One of the key roles here is played by the amygdala—the fear centre that was damaged in the reckless SM, whom we met in Chapter 2. The amygdala reacts strongly to oxytocin, which can moderate the activation of the amygdala in response to stressful situations, calming us down. This means that SM, with her damaged amygdala, would likely not benefit much from oxytocin sprays—at least not where fear was concerned. Oxytocin also reduces stress by acting directly on the HPA axis. The very neurons in the brain that kick off the HPA response carry receptors for oxytocin, and if the molecule binds to the receptor, it puts brakes on the activation of the HPA axis and the cortisol release. You feel less stressed—and stay healthy.

Such receptors for oxytocin are found not only inside our brains but all over our bodies. We have them in our bones, our hearts, even in our guts. It's hardly surprising, then, that plenty of studies have found links between levels of oxytocin and health. There is evidence that oxytocin has anti-inflammatory properties, that it promotes formation of new neurons in adult brains, that it reduces pain, and that it helps bone growth, potentially preventing osteoporosis. Oxytocin's effects are so powerful that some researchers have even dubbed it the "elixir of youth." If Ponce de León were still alive, he might consider his search over.

A direct proof of oxytocin's role in both sociality and health comes from voles (yes, those cute rodents again)—a proof that would be hard to obtain in humans for ethical reasons. In one study conducted at Florida State University, female voles were kept in isolation for four weeks. After the animals were released back into their group, the scientists noticed that not only were they more aggressive, their hearts were in far worse shape, too. Yet these effects could be reversed with simple injections of oxytocin.

Oxytocin may be the most studied neuropeptide linking our social lives with our health, yet it's certainly not the only one. There is also serotonin—the very hormone which has been discovered to be particularly abundant in the brains of tame Siberian foxes, and which has also contributed to the evolution of our domesticated species.

Unfaithful Mice and the Benefits of Massage

In the summer of 2014, the capital of Madagascar, Antananarivo, was hit by a swarm of locusts, consisting of billions of insects, flying in unison like a dark cloud of smoke rising above the houses. Similar plagues have been seen in Egypt, Israel, the American Midwest, and Australia.

At their most typical, locusts are not social creatures. They are loners. What makes them change into collective animals that may share close space with even ten billion others is the hormone serotonin.

Serotonin, also known as the "feel-good hormone," can not only make locusts more sociable—it can make humans more friendly, too. People who have higher levels of serotonin circulating in their systems are more cordial and agreeable. Even your success in speed dating may be affected by serotonin. When scientists followed over a hundred single Asian-American men who went on speed dates where each of the encounters lasted a mere three minutes, they discovered that those who had one particular variation of serotonin receptor genes had more luck—they were more likely to score a second date than those with another version of the gene.

While abundant serotonin causes us to be friendly, social isolation makes the levels of the neurotransmitter plummet, which in turn can prompt aggressive behaviours—an effect that has even been observed in lobsters. Serotonin has also been linked to blood pressure, Alzheimer's disease, pain perception, vascular tone, temperature regulation, and vomiting. In mice, serotonin can help regenerate the liver. In humans, low serotonin is associated with metabolic syndrome, a risk factor for heart disease. It has even been directly connected to longevity—at least in some animals, including mice and worms. One study of Japanese centenarians suggests there may be a link in humans, too. When researchers compared the serotonin transporter genes of those who've made it to at least a hundred to those of a younger control group, they discovered significant differences in how frequently one type of allele was present among the oldest people.

Just like with oxytocin, one way in which serotonin may be affecting our health is through its action on the HPA axis and on the production of the stress hormone cortisol, with more serotonin meaning, in general, less cortisol. In addition, serotonin can interact with oxytocin, each regulating the other's release, basically creating a feedback loop.

Another social neuropeptide, vasopressin, also interacts with oxytocin and orchestrates both our social lives and our health. Vasopressin is important for wound healing, kidney function, cardiovascular disease, and other functions. Unlike oxytocin, though, vasopressin seems more relevant to men. Also unlike oxytocin, it

appears that more vasopressin circulating in the body is not necessarily better, since it can elevate blood pressure and can make men
more aggressive. The likely reason for the hostile attitudes spurred
by vasopressin is that the hormone is very much about guarding
your loved ones from outside dangers. It can make rat mothers
fiercely protective of their babies, and make prairie vole males pos-
sessive of their mates. It can also make some animals ditch their
loose sexual habits altogether and become monogamous.

If you took cutesy pictures on greeting cards seriously, you might
conclude that mice make particularly devout partners. From
Valentine's Day to birthday cards, drawings of mice in love abound
in stationery stores across the world. Yet from a biological perspective, those images are off the mark: in many species of mice,
including your typical house mouse, both males and females swap
partners left and right.

But if you would like to turn a mouse monogamous, Romeo-and-
Juliet style, there is a way to do it, as long as you know how to insert
genes from one species to another. Back in the late 1990s, Larry
Young and his colleagues at the Atlanta lab took a vasopressin receptor gene out of prairie voles, those till-death-do-us-part-faithful
rodents, and popped it into the genomes of male mice, creating a
new type of transgenic animal. The new mice had a similar pattern
of vasopressin receptors in their brains to prairie voles, and behaved
in quite the prairie vole way as well: they were now more into huddling and grooming their female partners Hallmark-style.

In a similar fashion, by manipulating just one single vasopressin-
related gene, Young and his colleagues managed to make meadow
voles, which are as promiscuous as montane voles, more devoted
to monogamy. And although you can't exactly have your spouse
injected with prairie vole monogamy genes, studies do show that
vasopressin is also related to marriage quality in humans. A study of
Swedish twins revealed that in men, polymorphisms of one vasopressin gene in particular, called *AVPR1A*, can affect how well spouses

get on together—how often they kiss, how much they enjoy common hobbies, and how often thoughts about divorce cross their minds. For those who might be wondering: yes, you can order a genetic test for your future spouse to check his *AVPR1A*. All you need is a small vial of his blood, which you then send to a lab (for instance one in Temple City, California, provides such services). Whether doing so would be a good idea is another question—it might redefine the word "bridezilla."

An easier option for changing levels of vasopressin in human bodies to affect both health and behaviour involves small bottles with spray nozzles. In experiments, squirting vasopressin up people's noses has been shown to improve sleep and memory and to make women more conciliatory and men better at cooperation (the two genders tend to react differently to vasopressin—and sometimes to oxytocin, too). And just like the OxyLuv that I tested, you can order vasopressin nasal sprays on the internet. A bottle of Vaso-Pro sold on one website out of Hong Kong will set you back $69.99.

It may be quite tempting to order a container of OxyLuv and Vaso-Pro off the net and start spraying day in, day out. Please don't do that. Although such silver bullet solutions may be quite appealing, there are plenty of reasons why you shouldn't try to improve your longevity prospects by drugging yourself—or others—with non–FDA approved products (such sprays are for now only approved for use in lab experiments). We know extremely little about the long-term effects of oxytocin and vasopressin sprays, or their side effects. It's simply too risky. Luckily, though, you can boost the levels of your social hormones by using far safer measures. Like hugging.

Good animal moms have oxytocin-loaded kids. When mama rats engage in a lot of skin-to-skin contact with their babies, the little ones have increased concentrations of oxytocin in their blood. Humans are not much different: plenty of studies show that kissing, embracing, and even massaging raises oxytocin levels. What's more, the more oxytocin circulates in your blood, the more of it will be produced in the bodies of your children. Mothers and fathers who have high oxytocin are more responsive, more sensitive, and warmer toward their kids—hugging and kissing them more often, for example. So if you want your children to have higher levels of oxytocin, don't just hug them—hug your partner in parenting, too.

Back in antiquity, the Greek father of Western medicine, Hippocrates, claimed that "rubbing" was an important skill for any good physician to acquire. Contemporary research confirms that massages can boost oxytocin, leading to better health and, presumably, to longer lives. Same goes for other social hormones. Massage therapy can boost serotonin by 28 percent and dopamine by 31 percent. A massage with "a happy ending" works well, too—orgasms are quite good at raising oxytocin levels in the blood.

To get even more of the health-boosting and life-prolonging benefits of social hormones, don't just hug and massage your loved ones—do so while gazing deeply into their eyes. In a rather unsurprising finding, the more a mother looks at her baby's face, the more oxytocin gets pumped into her body. More remarkable was an experiment published in 2015 in the journal *Science*, which revealed that exchanging long gazes with your family pooch also boosts oxytocin levels—both in the dog and in the owner.

Simply spending time with others works well on your social hormones. When little mice are allowed to interact with other little mice in their nest, they grow up to have more oxytocin receptors in specific areas of their brains. Although, as far as I know, it hasn't been yet studied whether more playtime boosts oxytocin in human kids, there is evidence that after hanging out with their friends, adults have more oxytocin in their blood.

As for serotonin, you may have heard that stuffing yourself with foods abundant in the amino acid tryptophan, such as meat, will give you a serotonin boost, elevate your mood, and prolong your life. In reality, the meat-tryptophan-longevity link is a myth. Although it is correct that in experiments, giving people tryptophan supplements prompts them to produce more serotonin, and in turn makes them less irritable and quarrelsome, because of the way tryptophan is transported into the brain, foods containing tryptophan don't increase brain serotonin.

Luckily, you don't need to worry about your tryptophan intake—getting your serotonin from friendly back massages is completely safe and far more natural than taking pills. Our hominin ancestors didn't have access to either OxyLuv or tryptophan supplements—reciprocal grooming worked well enough for them.

⧗

The physiological connection between how friendly we are and how long and healthily we live makes perfect sense. After all, we have evolved this way. We have self-domesticated ourselves to be less aggressive and more trusting, more open toward others. As a result, our bodies have changed. Selection for higher levels of social hormones such as serotonin, dopamine, and oxytocin has left us with smaller jaws, flatter faces, and white eye scleras—and made our pink lips a simple reminder of how important social hormones were in the evolution of our species, and how much they can impact our bodies.

Today, social hormones are still the link between the quality of our friendships and family life on one hand, and our health and longevity on the other. They can explain why good marriage may equal good arteries and why having your best friend over reduces stress.

But as oxytocin, serotonin, or vasopressin go, we aren't all wired the same way. Some of us may carry the AA allele of oxytocin receptor gene *rs53576* and find it harder to get socially involved. Others may have the version of a vasopressin gene that makes working on a marriage an uphill struggle. But if that's the case for you, you certainly aren't doomed. You can still get more of the social hormones and their benefits by simply hanging out with your friends or hugging your family.

Yet these days many people ignore the many links between our minds and our bodies—our fight-or-flight response, our social hormones, the vagus nerve—and instead of investing in their relationships obsess about their diets and exercise. They skip gluten, load on turmeric, and religiously count their daily steps. Research shows, however, that a lot of this effort may be misplaced.

A FEW SUGGESTIONS TO BOOST YOUR LONGEVITY

To get a health-promoting increase of your social hormones such as oxytocin or serotonin, engage in more physical contact with others—kiss your partner more often, hold hands with your kids, hug your friends. Rub each other's backs. Treat yourself to a massage. And don't forget to look others in the eye—it may help raise oxytocin levels for both of you (and it works even if that "other" is a dog).

PART TWO

═══

HOW YOUR RELATIONSHIPS AND YOUR MIND CAN PROLONG YOUR LIFE

4

DITCH GOJI BERRIES

*Why Many Diet and Exercise Interventions
Matter Less than You Think*

IT WAS A SUNNY OCTOBER AFTERNOON in Vilamoura, a small town
on the Mediterranean coast of Portugal. It was warm, bordering on
hot, and the sweet scent of sun-heated olive groves lingered in the
air. With my bare feet I could feel several fallen olives scattered in
the grass. A yoga instructor, clad in purple leggings and a purple
tank top, was telling the class to move to a downward dog. I followed
her lead. I breathed in, I breathed out. In, out.

The days are well organized at the Longevity Cegonha Country
Club in Vilamoura, especially if you are taking part in their longevity
boot camp. After the yoga class there is Pilates, and later, a "Juices
and Water Detox" workshop and a stretching class. The weekly schedule is loaded with exercise, from tai chi to jogging, and healthy
eating courses. Each participant is offered personalized nutritional
coaching and can access an infrared sauna, a salt room, and a steam
room. The wellness area offers a "longevity ritual" (aromatherapy
massage), reiki, and even a dodgy-sounding "epigenetic test" that is
supposed to "provide clear information to help you implement a
food regime that will optimize your gene expression for wellness."

Everything in Vilamoura is centred on longevity—and I mean everything. In my room there was something called a "longevity soap" (according to the label) and a bag of some mysterious "longevity infusion," a kind of herbal tea. I was at the resort to do research, so I dutifully drank the tea. It tasted horrible, and I thought that if this was what long life felt like, I wasn't sure I wanted it anymore. The food at the resort's restaurant was far more appealing, albeit devoid of salt. For breakfast I got coconut milk porridge, a whole wheat bun, a slice of melon, some cheese, scrambled eggs with arugula, and a glass of freshly pressed mango-raspberry juice—no sugar added, the waitress assured me. For lunch, I ordered a "longevity salad" (lots of arugula, some quinoa, sunflower seeds) and a "longevity drink," which included cucumber and mint. Some boot camp participants, those on a detox program, got nothing but juice and soup. If you believe that eating well and exercising hard are the key to longevity, Vilamoura is certainly the place to be.

Yet the boot camp–goers of Vilamoura are certainly not alone in their obsession with nutrition and fitness—most Westerners these days seem to follow a similar philosophy. In their New Year's resolutions, over 80 percent of Americans say they want to change their diet or exercise regimen. As many as 45 percent buy organic foods and 70 percent drink low-fat milk. More than half take various dietary supplements, spending on average $56 a month. Even though less than 1 percent of Westerners have celiac disease, almost one-third of Canadians, 10 percent of Britons, and over 40 percent of Poles now try to eat gluten-free. We load up on protein, chase superfoods, and worry about omega-3s. And about our weight, of course.

If there is one longevity-related fear that seems particularly prominent across the Western hemisphere, it's that of excess pounds. According to one poll, most Americans think obesity is the most serious health concern faced by their country, and so they spend over $60 billion a year on weight-loss pills and slim-down diets. We seem truly obsessed with weight loss: just consider all the TV shows about it these days. There's *The Big Fat Truth*, *Extreme Weight Loss*, and *My 600-lb Life*.

I, too, admit to be slightly obsessed with staying the same size: I dutifully weigh myself each and every morning and feel slightly anxious on holidays when I don't have an easy access to scales. Here's the thing, though. For many of us, a few extra pounds may not be such a big deal after all. Not only does excess weight shorten lives less than does social isolation, but in certain circumstances, it may not even shorten lives at all. In the last two decades, research has accumulated on something scientists have dubbed the "obesity paradox": the fact that in many studies the plump and the pudgy come out better off in some aspects of health than do their slender counterparts. Take, for instance, advanced renal disease. If two patients, let's call them Mr. A (a slim guy) and Mr. B (slightly overweight), both have serious kidney problems and end up on hemodialysis, Mr. B has higher chances of surviving than does Mr. A. For every unit increase in BMI (body mass index), the probability of making it through hemodialysis increases by 10 percent.

A similar obesity paradox has been observed in cardiovascular disease. Let's say that instead of kidney problems, Mr. A and Mr. B end up with dodgy hearts. If the illness progresses to a full-blown heart failure, the slim Mr. A will be more likely to kick the bucket than Mr. B, whose risk of death could be even 12 percent lower than that of Mr. A.

The obesity paradox has been found in hypertension, in atrial fibrillation (a heart condition), and in lung-removal surgery. What's more, chubby people may overall live longer than the skinny of the world. Yes, you heard it right. By now we have quite a few papers published in top journals suggesting that being a bit overweight can add years to your life. People with BMIs between 30 and 35, which is grade one obesity and above the normal BMI range of 18.5 to 24.9, are 5 percent less likely to succumb to the grim reaper than the lean. It's only when your BMI tops 35 that your longevity potential starts to go considerably downhill.

One explanation for such counterintuitive results is that BMI is simply not a good measurement of how extra pounds affect health. If you are a classic "pear" shape, with relatively narrow waist but big hips, you may be far better off than an "apple" whose bulk accumulates in the belt area, even if your height-to-weight ratios are identical. Here is the reason: not all fat is created equal. A big belly, more scientifically known as "abdominal adiposity," in general means having too much fat stored around the internal organs, and this particular type of fat plays a role in inflammation and insulin resistance. On the other hand, the jiggly subcutaneous fat that accumulates under the skin in your thighs or around your hips is of a less troublesome quality (that's also the type of fat that helps women survive Donner party–type starvation).

Yet the issues with pear shape versus central chunkiness are still not enough to explain the obesity paradox. As for now, scientists are still unsure what the answer could be. Some suggest the paradox exists because people with weight issues tend to report concerns to doctors faster than do regular-sized folks. Others point to the properties of the fat tissue itself. For one, it can sop up toxins. Second, it can provide its "owner" with metabolic resources, which may be particularly needed in chronic disease—for instance in late-stage cancer. Obese people may also have altered levels of various substances circulating in their bodies, from cytokines involved in inflammation to some hormones—which could all play a role in the obesity paradox.

It appears that some of us, myself included, may be unnecessarily obsessed with the readings of our bathroom scales. What's more, many popular approaches to weight loss may reduce longevity. Consider high-protein diets. Although the jury is still out on whether they help shed unwanted pounds in the long term, research shows that too much protein can damage kidneys and shorten lives—something early Arctic explorers, including Vilhjalmur Stefansson, knew about very well.

Stefansson didn't look much like someone who had thoroughly explored the polar regions. With his slender build and longish hair, he more resembled a party-loving dandy than a tough adventurer who had lived for over a year on an ice pack. And yet his northern expeditions were what brought the Icelandic-Canadian his fame. It was also up north where he learned about the dangers of protein-loaded diets. In his writings, Stefansson described a phenomenon known across the Arctic as "rabbit starvation"—an illness caused by eating too much lean meat chock-full of protein, such as that of squirrels and rabbits. Here is what he recounted: "you are showing both signs of starvation and of protein poisoning. You eat numerous meals; you feel hungry at the end of each; you are in discomfort through distension of the stomach with much food and you begin to feel a vague restlessness. Diarrhea will start in from a week to ten days and will not be relieved unless you secure fat. Death will result after several weeks."

Although these days few people base their diets on little but squirrels, in those with chronic renal disease—and that's about 13 percent of the Western population—eating a lot of protein can accelerate the illness, so much so that scientists now advise against such diets in patients with chronic renal disease. What's more, there is some evidence that high-protein diets may harm kidneys even in healthy people. Authors of a study that revealed worrisome changes in renal function in young men who were put on a protein-rich regime concluded that those who follow such diets should have their kidneys regularly checked for abnormalities.

Faulty kidneys aside, upping your protein intake may generally shorten your life. Very low-carbohydrate diets may elevate the risk of imminent death by as much as 31 percent. While gorging yourself on protein might be a bad idea as longevity goes, another common

Western pastime, popping supplements, can bring with itself a whole other set of risks—even ones as serious as uncontrollable bleeding.

Beware of Supplements

A fifty-five-year-old Indian national living in Canada, let's call him Mr. Gupta, needed a coronary bypass. He wanted to have it done in his homeland, so he travelled all the way to Punjab, India, to have the surgery. At first, the procedure seemed to go well, but as time passed things started to go downhill in the operating room—Mr. Gupta just wouldn't stop bleeding. The doctors transfused one unit of plasma, then another. Several interventions later, the oozing finally subsided, but when the doctors checked the patient sometime after the surgery, they noticed his chest was covered in huge bruises—a rather disturbing photo of them can be now seen in a scientific paper the three cardiologists published in 2016 to document the case.

Later on, the doctors discovered the likely reason for Mr. Gupta's mysterious bleeding: his supplement pills. Before the surgery, Mr. Gupta was in the habit of taking three over-the-counter omega-3 and oleic acid pills per day, and a garlic-thyme supplement twice a day. Considering the effects such products may have on platelets clumping together to form blood clots, the doctors concluded they'd found the likely culprits. Mr. Gupta finally recovered, but his doctors commented in their later journal paper that the case "highlights the dangers of some dietary supplements."

Each year in the US alone there are an estimated fifty thousand serious adverse events connected to supplement consumption. In 2013, as many as 20 percent of cases of drug-induced liver injury were due to herbal and dietary supplements, up from 7 percent in 2004. What's more, those patients unlucky enough to have a liver failure after taking herbal pills are much more likely to require a transplant than are those who have damaged their liver by taking prescription drugs.

One supplement that is now making the rounds of the internet as a cure-all miracle is an extract from a Pacific islands plant called kava. It's supposed to work as a natural anti-anxiety medication, stop the growth of breast cancer tumours, treat depression, and protect you against Alzheimer's disease. The claims are wild, with basically no scientific evidence to support them.

What we do have evidence of, though, is that kava can damage the liver. Health authorities in several countries including Canada, the UK, and France have reported at least twenty-five cases of liver toxicity, including liver failure, after ingestion of kava. Products containing kava have been banned in some of these countries, such as the UK, while Consumer Reports placed kava on its list of "15 Supplement Ingredients to Always Avoid." Still, in some health junkie circles, kava remains highly popular. Across the US, well over a hundred specialized kava bars have opened in recent years, with more than fifty in Florida alone, offering juice-based and coconut water–based kava drinks.

So how can it be that something so innocuous-sounding as an herbal or dietary supplement can be so dangerous? First of all, about a quarter of supplements may have contaminants in them intro-duced in the production cycle—heavy metals, for instance, such as lead or mercury. Or pharmaceuticals. As of 2014, over five hundred supplements have been found to be tainted with pharmaceuticals, including amphetamine analogues or alprazolam (Xanax).

Second, we may simply not know how exactly the supplement works in the body. Prescription drugs have to undergo lengthy safety trials. Supplements don't. They are also practically unregulated—in the US, the FDA does not review their safety before they end up in shops. In the European Union, supplements are considered a "foodstuff," and their control is very difficult, especially consider-ing that many of them are sold online. In Canada, "natural health products"—vitamins, minerals, herbal remedies, and so on—must be assessed for safety by Health Canada, but the process is primarily paper-based, and the evidence submitted by manufacturers doesn't have to be particularly robust.

Another issue is that of drug interactions and side effects. Supplements are active substances and can interact with your prescription pills just the way regular pharmaceuticals do. And yet, one in six people who take prescription drugs also take at least one dietary supplement. To get into trouble you don't even have to go as far as the futurist Ray Kurzweil, the very same one who downs metformin to boost his longevity, who takes about ninety other pills a day, including green tea extract, echinacea, and gentian root. Two wrong substances mixed together can be enough to cause problems. St. John's wort, for example, can cause interactions with high blood pressure medications and with oral contraceptives.

Large, dangerous doses are also a common problem—both with herbal supplements and vitamins. Some toxic substances are basically poisons at high dosages yet beneficial to health in small quantities. This effect, known as hormesis, applies, for instance, to many phytochemicals, compounds that plants produce in order to kill or deter pests. Examples of phytochemicals likely known to many nutrition buffs include glucosinolates (behind the health benefits of broccoli) and tannins (red wine). Although it's basically impossible to overdose on broccoli due to the physical limits of your stomach— I challenge you to eat more than two or three heads—phytochemicals found in supplements are another story. Some green tea pills sold online in the US, for example, contain a minimum of 274 milligrams of phytochemicals called catechins per pill. The label says you should take three of these a day, which would bring you to a dosage exceeding what the European Food Safety Authority considers a liver damage risk.

Same thing goes for vitamin pills. High doses of vitamin C have been linked to renal failure, and high doses of vitamin E to cancer.

According to meta-analyses of studies, taking 400 IU or more of vitamin E per day can actually shorten your life, and so can beta-carotene supplements and vitamin A. Multivitamins aren't much better, either. In a study of over eighty thousand American physicians, those who took multivitamin pills had a 7 percent higher risk of dying from cardiovascular disease than those who didn't go for such supplements.

One reason for the damaging effects of vitamins may lie in the tricky workings of antioxidants in our bodies. Although often touted as quasi-miraculous substances that can wipe up dangerous free radicals and prevent aging, in reality the antioxidants that we swallow as supplements have much less rosy effects on our cells. More and more research suggests that free radicals are an important part of the body's repair mechanisms (that's why exercise is good for you—it produces free radicals). If you dump too many antioxidants in a purified form into your cells, they may end up disrupting these important repair processes. What's more, they can actually protect cancer cells from free radicals that are trying to get rid of the intruders. Just to be clear: this does not mean that antioxidants found in whole foods are bad for you. On the contrary. The reason for this goes back once again to the difference between mixtures of various naturally occurring compounds interacting with each other to your benefit (as in a carrot) versus purified components (vitamin pills).

If whole foods are much better for longevity than are supplements, maybe superfoods are super-good at boosting health? I decided to check it out. I ventured to a French equivalent of Whole Foods, Naturalia, about a twenty-minute drive from my house, taking with me a long list of supposedly extraordinary products advertised on blogs and in health magazines as superfoods. After spending far more money than I care to admit, I came home with a bag full of goodies. The next day was my superfoods day. For breakfast I whipped myself an organic Greek yoghurt with mixed berries, oats, and a generous sprinkling of goji berries, plus a cup of matcha and a glass of kombucha (fermented tea). Lunch was a kale and spinach smoothie with freshly pressed orange juice, fresh ginger, turmeric, and baobab powder. I also made myself a whole-wheat bread sandwich with chia seeds and ground flaxseed, topped with avocado and heirloom yellow tomatoes. I sipped some more matcha. For a snack, I had a beet and carrot smoothie with açaí berry juice plus two squares of dark chocolate—raw, of course. Dinner was Tuscan white bean soup with organic whole wheat pasta. And more kombucha. I was either going to turn into a superwoman or end up with a super-upset stomach.

I have to admit: at first I was quite pumped up. Just thinking of all these superfoods circulating around my body and perking up my cells made me feel energetic. As the day went on, though, I found myself craving cookies and fries. Like, I-can't-think-of-anything-else craving. What's more, by evening I was as tired as befits a working mother—basically the level of exhausted I reach on most days. Oh, well.

Of course, my experiment was extremely short and certainly could not qualify as anything scientific, not even close. Active substances in foods need time to do all their good work in our bodies, and one day is simply not enough. One could also argue that I didn't superfood myself sufficiently. Admittedly, the availability of superfoods in rural France falls short compared to, say, metropolitan US. There I could have also gone for moringa leaves, powdered durian fruit, manuka honey, ashwagandha powder, shilajit powder, Irish moss, or reishi mushrooms. My initial feelings of energy boost were quite likely the placebo effect at work. What I've also learned is that chasing superfoods takes a lot of effort and time—and money. And once I stopped whipping up baobab powder smoothies and started reading research studies and talking to scientists, I discovered that even if I did extend my superfoods day into a superfoods week or even a superfoods month, quite likely nothing much would change anyway. That's because most fancy superfoods don't really work.

If you are into longevity and health news, you may find it hard to follow all the headlines on superfood discoveries. I certainly do. One day it's goji berries, the next day it's matcha. What's all the rage right now, for example, is leaf powder from an Indian tree called moringa (*M. oleifera*). It's loaded with protein and iron, and is supposed to lower cholesterol, protect the cardiovascular system, and reduce inflammation. Hence moringa is being added to everything from nutrition bars and protein powders to juices and chips. Yet I couldn't find any reliable studies on moringa's health benefits. As one Canadian researcher has written, "The enthusiasm for the health benefits of *M. oleifera* is in dire contrast with the scarcity of strong experimental and clinical evidence supporting them." Same thing with goji berries, also known as the "Himalayan longevity fruit." Goji berries are supposed to treat diabetes, prevent cancer, and help with weight loss. Yet research on the fruit is beyond scarce. The vast majority of trials have been led by the same person, an employee of a company that produces goji juice. Talk about conflict of interest.

Another alleged miracle food, a yellow spice called turmeric, also doesn't stand up to scrutiny. Even though there do exist quite a few trials reporting benefits of its chemical component curcumin, most of them are erroneous signals. Curcumin has been classified as belonging to a group of compounds called "pan-assay interference compounds" (PAINS); when scientists screen chemical compounds looking for new drugs, pan-assay interference compounds tend to give false positive results because of their tendency to react with a wide variety of biological targets. A 2017 review published in the *Journal of Medicinal Chemistry* summed up the supposed miracle properties of curcumin quite simply as "much ado about nothing" and warned that the compound can "trick unprepared researchers into misinterpreting the results of their investigations." Curcumin is basically a "con artist" of the chemical world, showing false activity in poorly designed studies. So far no double-blinded, placebo-controlled clinical trial involving curcumin has been successful.

Just as adding fancy superfoods to your diet may not be the best idea, removing large groups of otherwise healthy products from your menu is also not the way to go if you want to boost your longevity. Even though the prevalence of celiac disease stays well under 1 percent in the US, a quarter of Americans say they avoid gluten. Among those, 35 percent do so for "no reason" other than the belief that gluten-free foods are somehow healthier. They are not. In one investigation of over 1,700 products available on the British market, researchers have found that gluten-free products such as breakfast cereal, bread, pasta, etc., tend to have more fat, sugar, and sodium than do their regular alternatives.

Other research has also found that they contain lower amounts of some vitamins. Instead, they tend to have more heavy metals. Blood and urine samples of people on gluten-free diets reveal they may have 47 percent higher levels of mercury and 80 percent higher levels of arsenic. To make foods without gluten, a great food texturizer, you need to process them more, often spiking them with additives. As a result, epidemiological research shows that people who habitually eat low amounts of gluten tend to have more diabetes and more coronary heart disease than those who eat more of it.

In general, if your diet excludes large numbers of items that are conventionally considered to be nutritious (fruits, vegetables, etc.), there is a good chance this diet is a fad. Before you ask—vegetarianism is not among them. For one, it only eliminates a single type of food, meat; but also, there is a substantial amount of research showing that going meat-free can significantly prolong your life. One study done in California has shown that vegetarians may live longer than others: an average of 9.5 years for men and 6.1 for women. Adding three ounces (85 g) of red meat to your daily diet, above what you normally eat, elevates the risk of death from cardiovascular disease by 16 percent over the next two to three decades of your life. If you exercise every day for twenty minutes to keep your heart healthy, that three ounces of bacon or steak may undo your entire effort.

If gluten-free eating doesn't make sense for most non-celiac people, if superfoods are not so super after all, and high-protein diets can hurt your longevity, then what should you eat to stay healthy? The answer is, I'm afraid, boring: lots of fruits and veggies. And they don't have to be exotic—so not rambutan or pitaya, unless you happen to live in southeast Asia. Just cabbage, tomatoes, broccoli, spinach, apples. The cheap, ordinary stuff. And you don't even have to go organic.

Is Organic Really Better?

In one 2014 interview, fashion designer Dame Vivienne Westwood suggested that people who can't afford to eat organic food should "eat less" rather than compromise their diets with conventional chow (unsurprisingly, she caused quite an uproar with that comment—people accused her of being elitist). Although most people aren't as adamant about organics as Dame Vivienne, over half of Americans now believe that organic food is healthier than its conventional counterpart. Scientists are not convinced. The results of studies on the nutrient content of organic versus conventional foods are mixed, with many showing no differences at all.

Take, for example, a trial in which a group of women consumed either 3.4 ounces (96 g) of organic or conventional tomato purée per day for three weeks, while their blood was monitored for concentrations of standard tomato nutrients: lycopene, beta-carotene, and vitamin C. The result? "No significant differences between organic and conventional exposures"—to quote the authors. Maybe the dosage was not enough? Well, in another study that had people eat 1.1 pounds (500 g) of apples a day for almost a month, there was also a nutritional tie between organic and conventional. One food not enough? In a Danish trial, sixteen people ate either a strictly controlled organic diet or conventionally produced equivalents for weeks at a time. Again, blood and urine tests showed no antioxidant benefits of any of the diets. Admittedly, there are a few studies that do show some small differences in favour of organic diets, yet in general these are not considered strong enough to warrant wide-ranging recommendations for organic eating.

Of course, abundance of nutrients is not the sole reason people choose organic—it's certainly not for me. Another big one is pesticides, or rather, the supposed lack of them in organic products. I'm saying "supposed" because organic foods do contain pesticides. There are many organic pesticides out there that are permitted for use in certified organic agriculture, such as copper sulfate or pyrethrum. Yet the fact that they are produced by nature—pyrethrum is a plant extract—does not mean they are necessarily less toxic than substances produced in a lab. In reality, we know very little about the long-term toxicity of organic pesticides. Yet as research progresses, some bad news on these compounds used in organic farming begins to surface. Chronic exposure to copper sulfate can result in liver disease, and in tests, pyrethrum comes out at least as acutely toxic as the infamous synthetic pesticide chlorpyrifos. Rotenone, meanwhile, another organic pesticide, ups the risk of Parkinson's disease by as much as eleven times.

What makes things worse is that we often simply don't know how much residue of organic pesticides can be found in organic foods. That's because authorities, such as the USDA, often don't test for them. Besides, some synthetic pesticides can be used in organic farming, too. In the US, twenty-five such products were approved at the time of writing. In an interview with the *Washington Post*, Nate Lewis, farm policy director for the Organic Trade Association, commented on organic eating: "It's critical you stop short of saying it's going to be healthier for you. We don't know that."

If you live in a country that has lax pesticide application rules, eating organic could make sense. But in places such as the US, Canada, Japan, or the EU, the regulations are so strict that even rule-exceeding levels of pesticides don't mean much. To establish safety standards for pesticides, scientists take the highest dose at which no harmful effects can be found in lab animals, and then divide it over and over. That's why the United States Environmental Protection Agency states on its website, "just because a pesticide residue is detected on a fruit or vegetable, that does not mean it is unsafe."

Many of the reports on pesticide danger tend to come from studies on farm workers and gardeners. And yes, if you are employed on a farm or you garden intensively, pesticides are something you should be concerned about, simply because it is possible to be exposed to far, far larger dosages than you may get from food. Pesticide applicators from Iowa and North Carolina who regularly deal with certain chemicals have double the risk of lung cancer. You should also be cautious using pesticides inside your home—that would be all these bug sprays against ants, cockroaches, and other creepy-crawlies. Applying such products four or more times per year may increase the risk of melanoma by 44 percent.

Once again, it's all about dosage. Some scientists go as far as to argue that synthetic pesticides, just like the natural ones we eat in fruits and vegetables (tannins in wine, glucosinolates in broccoli), may have a hormetic effect on our bodies—i.e., big doses are toxic, small doses are health-boosting. Meaning not only that tiny amounts of pesticide residues found in your food may not be harmful; they could even be beneficial. Although this controversial idea still remains to be tested in humans, some animal research does show that small doses of many supposedly toxic chemicals, including pesticides, can prolong life or reduce the incidence of cancer.

Here is a take-home message: if you have the financial means, sure, go ahead and pick up organic eats from time to time. I'm often tempted myself (better safe than sorry, right?). But the benefits of such foods, assuming they exist, don't justify our current obsession with everything organic. In the words of the American Cancer Society, "Vegetables, fruits, and whole grains should continue to form the central part of the diet, regardless of whether they are grown conventionally or organically."

If you must do something, buy foods produced in places such as the EU, the US, or Canada—places with strict pesticide checks. And simply wash your fruits and vegetables. Rubbing tomatoes under running water for only fifteen seconds removes almost 70 percent of some pesticide residues. Add lemon juice or baking soda to the wash water, and the benefits will be even more pronounced. But from a longevity perspective, it simply doesn't make sense to chase the purest foods. What's far more justified than organic food—and actually far more justified than superfoods, fad diets, supplements, worrying about a few extra pounds, or tracking your daily steps—is investing in your social life and in your mind.

The Roseto Effect

In 1960, Roseto, a small town in central Pennsylvania, seemed like an unremarkable place: neither particularly pretty nor charming, surrounded by unexceptional nature. Yet in seventeen years of practice in Roseto, the local physician, Dr. Benjamin Falcone, had barely seen any heart disease in locals under the age of sixty-five. That was highly unusual. When researchers compared Roseto to its surrounding communities, even ones sharing the water supply and medical facilities, they discovered that mortality rates in Roseto were 30 to 35 percent lower than in its counterparts.

It was not the genes, scientists soon concluded. It was not the diet, either. The Rosetans loved sugary treats, cooked with lard, and enjoyed sausages—41 percent of their calories came from fat. They made their own wine and loved to drink it—and did not abstain from hard liquor, either. What's more, the Rosetans also smoked and worked gruelling hours at a quarry or at a local factory. Obesity was common, too.

When the mystery was finally solved after years of research, the answer took many by surprise: Roseto's unusual healthiness was due to outstanding sociality, which had roots in the town's history. Roseto was settled in late nineteenth century by immigrants from Roseto Valfortore, Italy, who, though they forgot their healthy Mediterranean diets soon after settling, did not abandon their jovial attitudes. Surrounded by unfriendly neighbouring communities, from the very beginning the Rosetans felt they had to stick together. And so they did.

They looked out for each other, followed Italian traditions, and lived in multigenerational homes. Families were strong, elders were respected. They celebrated family events with big gatherings in their back gardens, with lots of food and plentiful wine, and did so often. The Rosetans believed individuals were part of something larger, a community—they had twenty-two civic organizations in a town of under two thousand inhabitants, from fishing and hunting clubs, sports clubs, and Christian youth organizations to a library.

Among Rosetan men, 81 percent were members of at least one such organization. Admittedly, women didn't have many clubs, but they were active in the town's social life through church groups and cooking—they gathered together often to prepare food for events and celebrations. The locals also cared for the looks of their town; they kept it clean and pretty, regularly picking up trash off the streets and planting flowers around the town centre. Last but not least, they were very neighbourly. In the words of one Rosetan housewife, "The neighbours were always in my kitchen and I was always in theirs. We talked. We knew what was going on there, and there was always someone around to help you and to keep you from feeling lonely."

Yet in 1963, a physician named Stewart Wolf, who studied extensively what became known as "the Roseto effect," made a dire prediction. Were the Rosetans to abandon their values and sociability, their healthiness would plummet and their mortality rates would start to resemble those in other small American towns. Unfortunately, that's exactly what's happened. As modernization set in and Roseto opened itself up to the rest of America, the community spirit evaporated.

Young people started dreaming the "American dream": bigger houses, fancier cars, more luxurious lifestyles. In the 1960s, the houses in Roseto were small and set close to one another, with little display of affluence—there was actually a social taboo against showing off wealth (it was considered bad luck). Now the new houses were being built suburban ranch-style: large and far apart. Driving replaced walking. People abandoned their community organizations and joined country clubs instead, as they strived to get ahead of the Joneses. In 1971, the town recorded its first heart attack in a person under the age of forty-five. Soon many more followed. Hypertension rates skyrocketed and so did general mortality. By the end of the 1970s, Roseto became a place like any other in the US.

You don't have to live in a Roseto-type place to experience the Roseto effect. A multitude of studies conducted around the world in both the twentieth and twenty-first centuries show very strong impacts of the mind and sociality on longevity. They show that if you want to change just one thing in your life, going for tons of fruits and vegetables in your diet may not be the highest priority. Instead, you should improve your relationships with others and work on your mindset.

Here are some stats: eating six or more servings of fruits and vegetables a day, versus zero, lowers the risk of mortality by 26 percent. Sticking to the famed Mediterranean diet means a 20 to 21 percent lower risk of dying within the next few years. The numbers for many social factors are much higher. A happy marriage equals a 49 percent lower mortality risk. Living with someone, even just a roommate, as opposed to living alone: 19 to 32 percent. Having a large network of friends: 45 percent. Other mindset and social indicators have effects similar to that of a super-healthy eating style: volunteering lowers mortality risk by about 22 percent—more or less as much as following the Mediterranean diet. If you were to add everything together, combining a good marriage, strong friendships, feeling of belonging, and so forth, to create a complex measure of social integration, or something that could be called the essence of the Roseto effect, you would get a whopping 65 percent reduction in mortality. And yes, as these numbers come from various studies done with various methods, they are hard to compare. But they still indicate some important trends.

Now, what about exercise? We certainly seem fixated on physical activity as a way to boost health—just look at the sales of various fitness trackers. One company, Fitbit, managed to sell 15.3 million devices in 2017, and as many as 20 percent of Britons use wearable technology to count their steps. In the US, one in six people use fitness bands and smartwatches. Whether all these exercise trackers actually work is another issue altogether. A study done in Singapore showed that using a Fitbit does not lead to improved health or fitness. Even more troubling was another trial in which wearing a fitness tracker actually led to slower weight loss.

Don't get me wrong: exercise is a good way to prolong life, there is no question about that. Just ask my family—I keep bugging everyone to do cardiovascular training. I have my reasons: research shows mortality reductions due to physical fitness in the range of 23 to 33 percent. And if you add several healthy lifestyle behaviours together—eating highly nutritious food, hitting the gym a few times a week, drinking in moderation, and not smoking—you can push your risk of death down by about 66 percent. That's a lot. That's also more or less the level of life extension you get from the Roseto effect, or from having a socially engaged and fulfilling life.

Imagine a Ms. A—a wellness junkie who dutifully attends her trampolining and Pilates classes several times a week, eats five or more servings of fruits and veggies a day, watches out for saturated fats, avoids sugar, and has never smoked. Now imagine a Ms. B—an overweight couch potato who loves cookies and chips and sometimes has a few shots of tequila too many.

Ms. A is also a slightly neurotic workaholic who feels like she is always running around. She is single, lives on her own and doesn't know her neighbours. She also doesn't have time to go out with friends and often feels lonely. She doesn't volunteer, and if you were to ask her about the purpose of her life she would be lost for an answer. On the other hand, our cookie-loving Ms. B leads a very socially engaged life. She has two very close friends and a loving husband, and often pops over to her neighbours' for a chat. She volunteers at a local charity and is very committed to its cause. She sings in a choir and does shopping for her elderly aunt once a week. She likes to sit on her porch enjoying sunsets.

Who will live longer? Of course, no one can ever predict the longevity of any particular person. But research that compares the effects of healthy eating and exercise on longevity to those brought by healthy social lifestyles shows that the lonely fitness freak Ms. A and the junk-food crazed yet very social Ms. B probably have a similar shot at becoming centenarians. That's the Roseto effect at play.

⧗

If you are obsessed with superfoods, organics, vitamins, and supplements, you can stop now. If you measure your daily steps with a fitness tracker and rush from one hyped exercise class to another, you can relax, too. And please don't freak out about every pound on your bathroom scales. From a health and longevity perspective these things matter far, far less than your social life and your mindset, and some of them can actually hurt your centenarian potential, not improve it.

My superfoods day made me realize how much time I would have to commit to chasing the best goji berries and following trends on the nutraceuticals of the day. And, according to research, I would be much better off spending that time playing Monopoly with my daughter or drinking coffee with my husband. My Portuguese longevity boot camp not only took precious days away from my family, it also cost money I could have donated to charity or spent on going out with friends. The hours I spend worrying about weight-loss strategies, I could commit to thinking about what matters to me in life or simply being more mindful. The supercentenarian Jeanne Calment didn't obsess about gluten or superfoods. She wanted to live life to the fullest, to savour it. I could try to be more like her, more optimistic. As a result, I might have a higher chance of living many healthy years. Maybe not 122, but perhaps ninety or ninety-five?

It would be truly great if you ate your five a day and did your two hours and thirty minutes of moderate aerobic physical activity a week. But you can also tackle your health issues from another direction: by investing more in your mind, in your friendships, and in your community. The effects might be even more pronounced than those of the best wellness-junkie lifestyle. What's more, easing up on nutrition and fitness obsession in favour of sociality and mindfulness could not only mean a life that is healthier, but also one that is more gratifying. A life worth living—something that no amount of kale or goji berries can give you.

Below you will find a table with an overview of studies showing the effects of different health behaviours on mortality. This can give you an idea of how much various things matter—or don't—for your longevity. The data comes mostly from large American samples, but not exclusively. Besides, many of the studies I've included here are meta-analyses (the gold standard in research). Keep in mind that you can always find one or two studies that will show very strong effects of some diet or other on mortality, or weak effects of social factors on the risk of death—but these studies tend to be either very small or poorly designed. Altogether the majority of evidence points to the greater importance of social integration and mindset to longevity than that of diet or exercise alone. This is why the World Health Organization now lists "social support networks" among its "determinants of health"—alongside the more widely acknowledged "balanced eating, keeping active," and "safe water and clean air."

Yet the mortality risk data presented in this chapter are not to be used as a strict guide to what's more important for longevity. Please don't try to evaluate whether five portions of broccoli a week are more important than two hours of volunteering. It's the general spirit that counts: being social and mindful affects health at least as much as do all of the traditional healthy lifestyle factors taken together.

The problem is, however, that in the twenty-first-century West, we all too often don't get enough of that close personal contact with others. With loneliness rates on the rise, some of us have to go as far as to pay $52 an hour so that professional "huggers" can provide us with a potentially life-extending oxytocin boost.

Tables 1a and 1b: Things that lower mortality risk (examples of studies).

Food/Exercise Intervention	Change in mortality risk	Social/Mind Intervention	Change in mortality risk
Exercise	-33% to -23%	Happy marriage	-49%
Fruits & Vegetables - 6 or more servings/day	-26%	Large social network	-45%
Whole grain intake - 3 servings/day	-23%	Feeling you have others you can count on for support	-35%
Mediterranean diet	-21%	Living with someone	-19% to -32%
Cruciferous vegetables intake—min. 5.8 oz/day	-20%	Extraversion	-24%
Being overweight	-6%	Volunteering	-22%
Omega 3s intake	no effect	Agreeableness	-20%
Vitamin C intake	no effect	Having a purpose in life	-17%
At least 4 healthy lifestyle factors combined (alcohol consumption, smoking, diet, physical activity)	-66%	A complex measure of social integration	-65%

Tables 2a and 2b: Things that increase mortality risk (examples of studies).

Food/Exercise Intervention	Change in mortality risk	Social/Mind Intervention	Change in mortality risk
Red meat intake	+29%	Loneliness	+26%
Obesity, grade 2 and 3	+29%	Pessimism	+14%
Vitamin A supplementation	+16%	Unhappiness	+14%
Beta-carotene supplementation	+7%	Neuroticism	+14%

A FEW SUGGESTIONS TO BOOST YOUR LONGEVITY

Ditch protein powders, expensive organics, and miracle foods (there are no miracles). Stop taking multivitamin pills—popping over for a chat in your neighbour's kitchen, Roseto-style, will bring you more health benefits, without the potential side effects. Skip fitness trackers—it's better to engage in some community gardening. If you are a bit overweight, stop obsessing: being social and mindful likely matters much more for your longevity.

5

THE GNAWING PARASITE
OF LONELINESS

Why Feeling All Alone May Shorten Your Life

THE "CUDDLING ROOM" I walked into resembled a cross between an undersized bedroom and a psychotherapist's office. It smelled of freshly washed floors and someone's lingering perfume. Right away my eyes drifted toward a pull-out couch dotted with pillows. It looked soft, inviting. I perched on its edge and took in the rest of the room: a small table with a box of hankies, some IKEA-style paintings, a shelf stuffed with books, and Buddhist-themed knick-knacks.

I have to admit: I was rather tense and uncomfortable, despite the easy demeanour of my personal "hugger," Katarzyna. She looked soft and, well, huggable. "Don't worry, everyone feels a bit weird the first time," she reassured me, asking me if I had a position in mind I'd like to start with. Before the visit I was sent a "menu" of cuddling positions I could choose from. There is the classic spooning position, one called "kitty" (in which the hugger sits on the couch while the client lies down with their head in the hugger's lap), and the "sailboat" (both lying down, the client with their head on the hugger's chest, the legs pulled up to cross the hugger's thighs). Some of the positions were simple, like the bear hug, while others, like the "paddle," looked as complicated as yoga. For $52 an hour I could choose how many cuddling positions I wanted, in whatever order my heart desired.

"Shall we start?" Katarzyna asked softly. She sat beside me on the couch and started smoothing out my hair, running her hand from the very top of my head down toward my shoulders. It felt awkward, very awkward. "Maybe let's lie down on the couch side by side," Katarzyna suggested. Once I was on my side, my face toward the window with Katarzyna behind me, I felt a tiny bit less weird (but still). She went on to gently pat my arm, then back to my hair. I felt very self-conscious. Although the website was very clear that the offer had absolutely nothing to do with sexual services, I kept worrying that I might have misunderstood something. But Katarzyna was professional, very massage-therapist-meets-psychologist. We kept chatting, which made the whole thing easier. Slowly, slowly, I began to relax. After a while, I had to admit it was actually quite pleasant, in a shampooing-at-a-hair-salon kind of way. My skin warmed up, and my heart slowed down. Oxytocin and serotonin must have been doing their job, making me calmer and healthier—and hopefully prolonging my life.

Warsaw's Salon Profesjonalnego Przytulania is the first professional hugging salon in Poland, and one of the very few such places on the planet. There is a professional cuddling centre in Portland, Oregon, one in Austin, Texas, and one "cuddlery" in Vancouver, Canada (same thing, different name). California already boasts many professional cuddlers. The idea is simple: if you are not getting enough hugs in your daily life, you can come to a cuddling salon for a fix. It's discreet, completely non-sexual, and quite likely effective at providing health-promoting oxytocin boosts. Katarzyna tells me that they have clients from all walks of life—young ones, old ones, middle-aged dads and twenty-something professional women. Some people come because their jobs leave them no time for social lives, and they want to feel a bit less alone in the big city. Others come because they want to get hugs they've never received from their mothers. Many come over and over again.

Cuddling shops may be quirky oddities, but judging from social isolation statistics, there seems to be a huge need for them. Considering the shrinking numbers of our friends and family, we can infer Westerners to be severely under-hugged. In Canada, the percentage of one-person households soared from 7 percent in 1951 to 28 percent in 2016. In the US, over a quarter of the population lives alone, too. That is still nothing compared to the European capital of solitude: Oslo, Norway. Here 52.9 percent of households are run by singles.

Of course, living alone doesn't necessarily mean not getting enough hugs or having low social support. But it might. Other stats support the view that becoming a professional cuddler may be a job of the future (and one unlikely to be stolen by robots, which is always a perk these days). In 2004, as many as a quarter of Americans didn't have even a single friend in whom they could confide. Recent years saw the average number of confidantes in our personal networks, including both friends and family, shrink from three people to two.

From a health and longevity perspective, that's disastrous. A large, high-quality study conducted in Alameda County, California, has shown that people who score low on social integration—have few friends and relatives, aren't married, and don't belong to community organizations—are as much as three times as likely to die over the next seven years than those blessed with close-knit relationships. You might think that such effects of friends and family on longevity might only apply to seniors. It could be, after all, as simple as having someone check up on you regularly to make sure you haven't fallen down the stairs and broken your hip. But that's not the case. It's been shown over and over that people of any age who have poor social relations suffer more heart attacks, strokes, diabetes, and even pregnancy complications—hardly something regular family visits could prevent.

The positive effects of social capital on longevity are not simply due to wellness-related reminders from your loved ones, either—to mothers, brothers, and besties talking us into eating better, exercising more, or giving up those stinky cigarettes. Although people who share accommodation with another person tend to eat a larger variety of fruits and vegetables, in general their diets don't differ all that much from those who are lonelier. Also, things like nicotine habits proliferate in social circles. Some people find it simply too hard to resist a smoke if their friends light up.

Admittedly, there is one way in which reminders and nudging by friends and family clearly do contribute to longevity: compared to loners, people who are surrounded by caring others are over three times as likely to listen to their doctors and take their pills as prescribed. But this, too, is not enough to explain the staggering influence our interpersonal relationships have on our health. In epidemiological studies, controlling for patient compliance with medical treatment is the norm, and yet, the effects persist. What's more, fascinating lab research provides additional evidence that the links are not merely cultural or behavioural, but also physiological.

Imagine over three hundred people coming into a research lab and getting voluntarily infected with cold viruses squirted directly into their nostrils (the motivation must have been the $800 each person was paid for participation). During the month before the infection, the volunteers received six phone calls from the researchers on six separate days, during which they were queried on their social interactions on each day. With whom did they hang out? For how long? Was it pleasant? Then, after the virus-squirting exposure, the brave volunteers were kept in quarantine for five days and were repeatedly assessed for cold symptoms (for instance, their used hankies were weighed for "nasal secretions"—also known as snot).

When the results came in, a clear picture emerged: loners had a 45 percent higher risk of developing a cold than did more gregarious people, even though everyone was exposed to the exactly same dose of the virus. In other words: hanging out with your friends can protect you from sniffles.

The biological links between our social connections and health are, once again, largely due to the interplay of neuropeptides such as oxytocin, dopamine, endorphins, and serotonin, as well as the HPA axis. Sometimes, though, they can be far more straightforward. When scientists compared the gut microbes of wild baboons, they discovered that the closest buddies had the most similar gut microbiomes—just like Aura Raulo's mice in the forests of Oxfordshire. And since healthy gut microbiome has been linked to a lower risk of cancer, heart disease, diabetes, and so on, such microbiome-diversifying exchanges between friends could boost longevity. Of course, social contact can also function as a route for parasites and deadly pathogens. As Raulo tells me, finding balance between healthy microbe-diversifying transmissions and escaping risky transmissions is a challenge social animals deal with all the time.

Although having physical contact with others, as well as being integrated in the community—meeting friends, being married, participating in clubs—are vital to our health and longevity, the objective quality of our relationships is only a part of the story. What matters almost as much is what we think about our social lives, how we perceive them. On paper, you may seem to be doing well in the friendship and family department, but if you consider yourself lonely, your centenarian potential will suffer nevertheless.

Preventing Gangrene, Messing Up Sleep

Lindsay, age thirty, realized she was lonely when she became a mother. "I would stand in front of the window looking out over the neighbourhood . . . and I would think about how everyone was sleeping . . . and I felt like I was the only one awake feeling my wretched feelings." Dani, age thirty-two, says loneliness means not feeling human. "I feel small and curled up, like a tiny animal in permanent hibernation. Nothing gets through and everything's cold." To Daniel, age eighteen, loneliness is like a parasite. It "lives in my stomach constantly, and I can feel it eating all my organs with each week that passes."

The quotes above come from a website called the Loneliness Project, founded a few years back by Marissa Korda, a twenty-five-year-old graphic designer in Toronto. The landing page is laid out as an apartment block, awake despite the darkness of night, the sounds of busy urban life rising from an invisible street below. In the building's windows, black silhouettes of people can be seen, one per apartment—reading books, working on computers, or just gazing at the world outside. If you click on them, a window will pop up with a person's name, their age, and their accounts of loneliness. The images are made up, but the stories are real—stories of not fitting in, of seclusion, of not being understood by anyone. They are submitted to the website by readers and three stories are posted per week. Although they differ in their content, they all make for a heartbreaking read.

Scientists say loneliness and social isolation are two distinct concepts. The first one is subjective (you feel like there is no one out there for you—no friends, no family, no romantic partner, no caring neighbours), the second one is objective (there really is no one out there for you). You may be surrounded by family and friends, and yet feel lonely. On the flip side, you may be truly alone—think cabin in the Alaskan wilderness—and not experience the parasite of loneliness. But just as is social isolation, loneliness is prevalent in the Western world. One in five Canadians claims to be lonely, while in the US, the number of people reporting loneliness is around 17 percent. Western Europe seems a bit better off, with rates of loneliness hovering around 10 percent. With old age, loneliness rates climb almost everywhere across the globe. In Canada, approximately 50 percent of seniors over the age of eighty say they are lonely.

All that is bad news, since it's not only objective social isolation that matters for health and longevity. Subjective feelings of loneliness are important, too. One 2015 meta-analysis of studies established that while objective social isolation may increase the risk of death by 29 percent, reported loneliness ups it by 26 percent. And if you are both objectively alone and subjectively feel alone, your odds of becoming a centenarian go downhill even more, since the effects of isolation and loneliness are cumulative. If you add up multiple positive indicators of social support, objective and subjective, it may all increase your chances of survival by a whopping 91 percent. Eating organic goji berries and doing push-ups doesn't come anywhere close in giving you this kind of longevity boost. As for specific health effects, loneliness appears to push up the risk of cardiovascular disease, stroke, and even urinary incontinence. And, of course, it can also shorten life rather dramatically by suicide.

However, here's one thing about loneliness: it used to be good for us. In fact, we have likely evolved to feel lonely from time to time. John Cacioppo, a University of Chicago neuroscientist who was so focused in his career on the study of loneliness that he was jokingly nicknamed "Dr. Loneliness," liked to compare loneliness to hunger and thirst. Just like the two latter states, he claimed, loneliness is a signal that something has gone awry in our lives, something that we should change, fast. When we are hungry, we should look for food. When we are lonely, we should seek connection with others.

For our ancestors, the particular biological changes brought by feelings of loneliness may have actually helped with longevity—I'm talking about the times when your centenarian potential was most likely to be ruined by sabre-toothed cats, not diabetes. When our forefathers and foremothers were left on their own, without their tribe, the feeling of loneliness activated a whole set of physiological changes aimed at survival. Imagine you are living fifty thousand years ago somewhere on the African savanna. You have a disagreement with your fellow tribespeople and they kick you out. You are on your own. The squabbling may be over, but now you are at risk of becoming a lion's next meal. You run around looking for a place to hide, and as you do so, you get scratches all over (those thorny acacias can be a nuisance). If you do get into a scuffle with a predator, and you somehow get out alive, you may have even more scratches and wounds that will soon start teeming with bacteria. To survive, your body needs to start fighting the infection—and it better be efficient.

When we feel lonely, Cacioppo once told me in an interview, our immune systems switch away from fighting viruses toward a better antibacterial response. In a tribe, viral infections spread easily, so the body has to be ready to take them on. But once a person is secluded, the risk of a virus goes down, while the risk of lion-induced wounds teeming with bacteria goes up, and that's what the body focuses on. Just as the feeling of hunger turns on your search for food and puts your body in an energy-saving mode, your feeling of loneliness switches on your "alone on a savanna survival mode." Such a turn away from an antiviral response toward an antibacterial one means that when you feel lonely, inflammatory activity in your body goes up. Circa 50,000 BCE, it could have prevented you from losing limbs, or your life, to gangrene, but circa 2020 it just raises your risk of metabolic syndrome.

Another biological consequence of loneliness is troubled sleep. If you are all alone on the savanna, succumbing to deep slumber is not a good idea (it makes it too easy for lions to creep up on you). In his lab studies, Cacioppo found that lonely people experience more fragmented and restless sleep, even if they sleep for as many hours as those who don't feel all alone in the world. That, of course, is bad news for your health—poor sleep can mean heart disease, diabetes, and cancer, and ultimately result in a shorter life.

The UK is the most sleep-deprived country in the world, with 37 percent of Britons claiming they don't get enough z's. Canada and the US place third, right after Ireland. For that sad state of affairs we tend to point fingers at crazy work schedules and smartphones. But maybe the fact that we feel so under-slept can also be blamed on the spreading epidemic of loneliness, which makes our hominin bodies all jumpy at night in case hungry lions sneak into our bedrooms. We simply don't sleep well because our lonely bodies are in savanna survival mode.

But loneliness is not just about troubled sleep or increased inflammation—there is also the simple stress of it. The closest I've ever been to the "alone on the savanna" scenario was when I walked across a national park in Tanzania with a local guide—just me, the guy, and my husband. The guide had a shotgun, yet my heart was still pumping fast, cortisol sloshing in my veins. What if I got lost and was abandoned there? At night? No, thank you. I felt very far away from my "tribe" (family and friends), and wished that our group was larger than just the three of us. I could clearly feel in my own tensed-up body how evolution discourages aloneness. It's no wonder that lonely people tend to have increased activity of the HPA axis and elevated cortisol levels. You can see it in their saliva—the very next morning after a day filled with loneliness people have more cortisol in their saliva right after they wake up. Ready for fight or flight— perfect in case they open their eyes to a breakfast-ready carnivore staring them down.

In our evolutionary past, the pangs of loneliness may have served to save our lives. They induced a beneficial anti-wound and anti-pred-ator biological response and made us hunger for connection, so that we would go back begging for forgiveness and inclusion. In the past, loneliness tended not to last long. You either re-connected with others or you got eaten by something. These days, though, the feel-ing of loneliness is no longer so adaptive. "When we remain lonely in a contemporary society for long periods, the costs start to outweigh the benefits," Cacioppo told me. Poor sleep leads to obesity, heart disease, and diabetes, accelerates tumour growth, and shortens life. Inflammation damages tissues and contributes to cancer. Elevated cortisol messes up your immune system and blood pressure.

But that's not the end of it, unfortunately. To find out more about the costs of chronic loneliness and what exactly happens to the bodies of contemporary humans who get kicked out of their "tribe," scientists study something they call ostracism.

Shunning, Banning, and Computer Games

For Robin Thompson, the fear of being ostracized, or excluded from her community, was so great she had suicidal thoughts and developed agoraphobia. "It was very hard for me to leave the house. I would get in my car just to go to a grocery store and I would get to the end of the street and just have to turn around and come back," she recalls. Her panic attacks got so bad one landed her in a hospital. She was convinced she was having a cardiac arrest.

Although Thompson was born a Jehovah's Witness, a daughter of an elder no less, she started having doubts about the religion in her teenage years. "But you are not allowed to question anything. That can be dangerous. You have to suppress these doubts; you can't talk about them with other Jehovah's Witnesses," she says. The danger here is that quitting the religion—or "disassociating" yourself, as it is known—almost automatically brings with it shunning by the rest of the community. They stop talking to you. They pretend you no longer exist.

Years passed and Thompson got married, yet her doubts didn't subside. In 2006, she and her husband gave up on the religion for good, but weren't ready to officially announce their disassociation. They did so two years ago, after they started posting videos on YouTube denouncing issues within the religion. The shunning followed. "I went over to talk to my parents, and it was like they were different people. It was very robotic, the way they spoke to me, and very matter of fact: 'Well, we love you. And we will miss you. But we can't have anything to do with you anymore,'" Thompson says. Being excluded from the community meant losing her friends and her network of support. "You feel like your entire family died in a horrible accident, yet you know they are still alive. It's an incredible sadness and loneliness," she says. The shunning has also likely taken a toll on her immune system and physical health, Thompson says. Even though beforehand she could go years without a cold, in the few months after being shunned she had no less than five flu-like infections. She also says that she suffers from "a lot of pains and aches," despite being just forty-five.

Jehovah's Witnesses is certainly not the only religion that practises shunning: it's also known in Scientology, orthodox Judaism, and Catholicism. Under the name of ostracism, exile from a community was commonly used as a penalty by ancient Greeks. The citizens would vote on which disliked person to kick out of their town by writing that person's name on *ostraka*—shattered fragments of pottery. Luckily, though, contemporary scientists don't have to resort to writing their subjects' names on broken IKEA mugs and shunning them for years in order to study the effects of ostracism. A simple computer game will suffice.

The game is called *Cyberball* and it works like this: you are told you are going to play online. Your goal is to catch and toss a virtual ball with two other participants, whom you won't see (they are supposedly sitting glued to their own computer screens). You don't know the other people, and they don't know you. *Cyberball* is no *Grand Theft Auto* with its stunning graphics—it features just three roughly sketched figures throwing a ball around. The secret here is that the other players aren't real. They are just part of the program, designed to either make you feel included or ostracized. If scientists want to make you experience rejection, the other "players" will pass the ball to you a couple of times, then start acting as if you weren't even there, playing only with each other. In the scenario where you are to feel included, the little cartoon people will keep tossing the ball to you throughout the whole game.

By now over five thousand people have been made to feel either ostracized or socially included using *Cyberball,* and their psychological and physiological responses measured in dozens of ways. One fascinating finding to emerge is that the pain of loneliness is not a mere metaphor—it's real. In one experiment, researchers asked volunteers to play *Cyberball* while inside a magnetic resonance imaging scanner. As some of the participants got sidelined by their virtual ball-tossing buddies, scientists noticed that an unexpected area of the volunteers' brains kept lighting up—the very same one that would light up if someone punched them in the gut. In other words, social pain activated neural networks that normally respond to physical pain. The hurt of romantic breakups and friendship squabbles, it appears, could be as real as toothache.

Further *Cyberball* studies have shown that some people are more susceptible to the pain of loneliness and social rejection than others. Carriers of the GG variant of the oxytocin receptor gene *rs53576* feel more gloom if they are ostracized than do those with the AA genotype. It's hardly surprising—after all, GG people are generally the more empathic and socially sensitive types.

Yet it's not just our genes that affect our propensity to experience the parasite of loneliness. It works in the other direction, too, with loneliness changing our genes. Some of the most affected ones are the pro-inflammatory genes, which are overexpressed in people who perceive themselves to be particularly excluded—their genes are working harder than average to convert instructions from the DNA into products such as pro-inflammatory cytokines. In one fascinating but disturbing study, scientists collected reports on loneliness from 181 people. Years later, once all these people had died, their bodies, which had been donated to research, were studied. The results showed that as many as 380 genes had worked differently in these lonely people, most of them in overdrive—genes associated with the immune response, Alzheimer's disease, and cancer.

Being lonely doesn't just gnaw at your soul, apparently. It damages your body, too, all the way down to your genes. To boost your health and prolong your life, you'd be better off without this unpleasant feeling—and sometimes all you need is a warm shower.

A Cup of Hot Chocolate

On November 5, 1981, at 5:21 p.m., nineteen-year-old Lisa D'Amato, clad in a bathing suit, turned on a shower in her dorm at the State University of New York at Binghamton and stepped under the spray. Ten hours later she was still in there, drenched in water, asleep on a rubber mattress. By November 9, her feet were full of wrinkles, but she wasn't ready to stop showering. D'Amato finally turned the water off on November 10, her shower lasting a world record 121 hours and one minute.

D'Amato might have attempted the extra-long shower for charity reasons (she was raising money for the American Cancer Society), but studies show that in everyday life people take prolonged showers when they feel lonely, rather than charitable. The first such report came in 2012 when two Yale University researchers calculated that people who consider themselves socially isolated take more warm baths and showers. What's more, by now plenty of other data has connected our feelings of loneliness with physical temperature. Imagine, for example, that you are eating dinner in your kitchen. How warm is the room? Curiously, your answer will likely depend on whether you are dining alone or surrounded by friends or family. In one experiment, researchers approached dozens of people who were lunching at a food court and asked them to estimate the temperature of the building. Those who ate on their own said, on average, 68.3 degrees Fahrenheit (20.21°C), while those who ate with others guessed 72.6 degrees (22.57°C). In reality, it was 70.7 degrees (21.5°C), somewhere in the middle. In other studies, scientists obtained similar results: the differences in temperature perception are not huge, but they are clearly there.

And if you want to save on heating, you could try thinking of your loved ones more often. Such recollections can make people estimate the room temperature as higher than it really is by as much as 3.6 degrees Fahrenheit (2.0°C). Even a hot cup of tea or coffee can change our perceptions. Holding a steaming drink in their hands makes people more trusting and "warm" toward fellow humans.

Although the connections between our feelings of social inclusion and physical temperature may seem coincidental, there is a biological explanation for why they should exist. It all boils down to the fact that animals are economical creatures for whom saving energy is a high priority. Consider emperor penguins. In July, when the Antarctic winter hits its coldest and the temperatures plunge below –49 degrees Fahrenheit (–45°C), male emperor penguins stand patiently trying to hatch their precious eggs. They don't go anywhere, they don't hunt, and they don't eat. They may fast for as long as 115 days, yet have to keep their egg warm and cozy—and they have to survive themselves despite the brutal cold. To do so, they huddle. Tens of thousands of these large birds may squeeze together on patches of snow the size of a football field, elevating the temperature inside the pack to 99.5 degrees Fahrenheit (37.5°C). If emperor penguins didn't huddle, their individual fat stores wouldn't allow them to survive the chilly Antarctic winter and hatch the eggs. They would all starve to death.

For many animals, huddling allows them to save precious energy resources. In some species, it can lower an individual's basal metabolic rate by more than 50 percent. That, in turn, ups chances for survival—the creatures need less food and can endure wintry temperatures. Our ancestors weren't much different. By huddling through chilly days, they warmed each other up, keeping the body surface area exposed to the elements as small as possible. What was important, though, was to know whom you could trust to keep you warm on a cold night. The better a "friend" someone was, the more you could count on them to snuggle up with you.

Throughout evolution, this connection between social relationships and physical warmth became hard-wired in our brains. Today, the mechanisms that regulate body temperature and those that determine how "warm" or "cold" we feel toward other people tend to overlap. The key lies in the insula, a small, pyramid-shaped structure deep within the cerebral cortex that is important both for how we perceive temperature and how we perceive others. Animal studies also suggest that oxytocin may play a role. Mice that don't have receptors for oxytocin have trouble regulating their body temperature.

What that all means for us modern humans is that our bodily thermostat can serve as a clue to how well connected we are socially. Do you crave hot showers? Do you suddenly feel chilly even though the room temperature is objectively quite cozy? Maybe your body is telling you to get in touch with your close ones to get your oxytocin boost.

On the other hand, playing with temperature can help you deal with the feelings of loneliness and exclusion. In Agatha Christie's *The Mysterious Affair at Styles*, a wealthy old woman, Mrs. Inglethorp, quarrels with her husband. "You have lied to me, and deceived me," she exclaims. After the fight, Mrs. Inglethorp retreats to her boudoir and complains to her maid of "great shock" and betrayed trust. The maid offers a simple solution: "You will feel better after a nice hot cup of tea, m'm."

The maid was on to something when she claimed that a hot drink can lift your mood when you are upset after a fight. It can be hot chocolate, it can be tea—it doesn't matter what drink it is as long as holding it warms up your hands. In a similar fashion, curling up by a fire or indulging in a long, steamy shower may potentially reduce loneliness.

The problem, however, is that while hot chocolate or a bath may temporarily lift us out of the misery of being all alone, it's just a temporary fix, a bit like treating a headache with Tylenol without addressing any underlying medical causes. If you are chronically lonely, what you need for a true health and longevity boost is to get rid of the feeling for good—and for that even a 121-hour hot shower wouldn't be enough. Banishing loneliness requires far more effort and is unfortunately an uphill battle, since feelings of isolation change the way we behave and think, trapping us in a catch-22.

Loneliness Habits and Magic Mushrooms

In a laboratory room at the University of Central Lancashire, UK, an eighteen-year-old student was seated in front of a laptop, a weird contraption attached to his head, something like a *Star Trek* Vorta command headset. Yet this was no sci-fi invention. It was an eye-tracking device used by psychologists and neuroscientists to study what attracts our attention. By analyzing data coming from cameras and mirrors mounted around the eye area, researchers can measure gaze direction and eye movements to better understand how visual information is processed in different situations by different people.

On that particular day at the University of Central Lancashire, the eye tracker was being used to study what happens when lonely people face socially unpleasant situations. Just after each of the dozens of students who volunteered for the project installed themselves in front of the laptop, they were presented with eight video clips, each lasting a mere twenty seconds. Two videos would play at the same time, show-ing people in different social situations—either positive ones (smil-ing or nodding at one another) or threatening ones (turning their backs on each other, ignoring each other). Since the researchers also surveyed each participant on their level of loneliness, they could weight this data against the measurements from the eye tracker. Here is what they found: people who were particularly lonely paid far more attention to threatening social situations than did those who felt happy with their relationships—the lonely subjects' eyes would automatically drift to images of shunning and disdain.

A similar picture emerged from other studies, including those using functional magnetic resonance imaging: loneliness makes us fixate on social threats. Is this guy sneering at me? Is that girl giving me the cold shoulder? In Cacioppo's studies, lonely people could pick up on negative social signals within 120 milliseconds, less than half the time it takes us to blink. This obsession with social threats makes relationships an uphill battle for lonely people, who tend to withdraw from social situations and distrust other people. They feel a hunger for connection, yet if that hunger is not satisfied soon and becomes chronic, they start growing a thick, thorny skin to protect themselves from potential hurt.

"In 120 milliseconds you are not doing that deliberately. Your brain is on hyper-alert even when you are just sitting and resting," Cacioppo told me. Once again, such behaviour made sense on the African savanna. You wanted to be vigilant in case members of some other tribe were out to get you with their sharpened sticks. Loneliness makes our brains react differently to strangers versus people we know well: it turns on "hunger" for reconnection when we see those we know, but not when we face outsiders. Such fixation on "stranger danger" was a good idea when we lived in small groups, but not in our large, modern society, when making new friends could help overcome solitude.

Although this may all sound bleak if you are among the millions of Westerners who feel chronically lonely, the good news is that understanding the mechanisms of loneliness can set you on the path out of it—and protect you from its health-damaging consequences. According to Cacioppo, the first and foremost step is changing your mindset about loneliness. "Knowing that there isn't something wrong with you, but rather that it's a biological response designed to help you. It's not that you are unlovable, it's just the lonely state trying to promote self-preservation," he told me.

To reduce loneliness you don't have to jump head-first into a whirl of partying and networking, and you don't need to sign up for dozens of dating portals and friendship-making apps. Here's what you can do. First, stop blaming yourself—loneliness is natural and perfectly normal. Humans have always experienced it and always will. Simply recognizing that loneliness is not a genetically-based sentence or a result of life trying to get you can push many people out of being lonely. The second step is to try to change the way you look at others, to realize that the distrust and hostility you may be feeling is likely just your savanna-evolved body prepping you for an attack by an enemy tribe.

Unless an attack by an enemy tribe is something you may realistically fear in the near future, a cognitive behavioural therapy might be a good idea. Finding a professional therapist could work well, but you could also try changing your thoughts on your own. In his book *Loneliness: Human Nature and the Need for Social Connection*, Cacioppo describes techniques for consciously stopping negative thoughts: "'Is it literally true that everybody hates me? No? Then why do I keep saying this to myself? Let's recognize the habit, and the harm that it causes, then stop it.'" This is followed by redirecting them in a more positive way: "'Yes, I'm not as sociable as I would like to be, but that's a far cry from "Everybody hates me." Some people actually like me.'"

For a more radical approach, you could try hypnosis—if people are hypnotized and their thoughts are redirected toward feelings of social connection, their loneliness tapers off. And if that still doesn't work, there are also magic mushrooms. And yes, that recommendation is actually science-tested. In one experiment conducted in Switzerland and published in the prestigious journal of the National Academy of Sciences, after taking psilocybin, an active compound of magic mushrooms, volunteers reported feeling less socially excluded—and the effects were also confirmed by functional magnetic resonance imaging scans of their brains. According to one of the study's authors, psilocybin might have real potential for the treatment of severe loneliness. You could enjoy psychedelic euphoria, feel less isolated, and increase your centenarian potential in one go. Just keep in mind that for now taking psilocybin is illegal in many countries, the US, Canada, and the UK included—so to profit

from its loneliness-busting effects you would have to volunteer for
another scientific experiment. Or simply wait a bit—it may soon
become legal. Two US cities, Oakland and Denver, have recently
decriminalized possession of magic mushrooms (although commercial sales still remain illegal).

⧖

Loneliness kills—and not just because it can drive a person to suicide. It kills slowly by messing with your stress response and altering
the functioning of your genes. Feeling all alone in the world may
have nothing to do with how many friends you have or how much
they care about you, but it can still up your risk of cancer and heart
disease, and it can shorten your life more than obesity or a couch-
based lifestyle.

In the Western world, as many as one in five people experience
loneliness. It hurts them just as much as physical pain does, like a
gaping wound. They may feel so desolate that to get an oxytocin
boost, they sign up for sessions at professional cuddling shops. They
may take particularly long and hot showers to fool their brains into
feeling socially connected. These measures do work, but only temporarily. To avoid the negative health consequences of loneliness,
lonely people need to realize that the feeling is natural, that we've
evolved to have it. It used to protect us, yet now it often leads us
astray, locking us into negative patterns of thinking. With effort,
behavioural therapy, or even hypnosis, such patterns can be changed.
The feeling of loneliness can be decreased even if you don't make a
single new friend.

But subjective social isolation, albeit important, is only part of the
story. The objective part—how many close, loving relationships we
have—matters at least as much for our longevity and health as does
the subjective feeling of loneliness. What we need is what scientists
call a "strong social support"—a network of friends, family, and

neighbours to whom we can turn in times of need. But how can we be sure we have enough of that social support? And if we don't have enough of it, how do we know whether we've slipped into the "socially isolated" category? Is having one close friend enough? Or are three or more friends necessary if you really want to increase your centenarian potential? Do you have to be married to reap the longevity benefits? Luckily, we have decades of research to give us some answers, starting with a simple tip: if you want to stay slim, don't roll your eyes.

A FEW SUGGESTIONS TO BOOST YOUR LONGEVITY

If you feel lonely, the first step is to realize that this is a biological adaptation and not a sign that something is wrong with you. Stop blaming yourself. Try to change your thought patterns. Think, "Yes, I'm not as sociable as I would like to be" instead of, "Everybody hates me." Try to warm yourself up physically—take warm showers and drink hot tea. Don't fixate on social threats or how others are "trying to get you."

6

FRIENDS WITH
(LONGEVITY) BENEFITS

How Marriage and Friendships Prolong Life

"NO! PLEASE DON'T EAT ME! I have a wife and kids—eat them!"—cries Homer in one of the episodes of *The Simpsons*. Although throwing your spouse to a bear or a cannibal is certainly one way in which marriage could prolong your life, it's not the only one. Married people have lower risks of heart issues, cancer, and Alzheimer's disease. They even sleep more soundly and respond better to flu vaccines. If a married person does have a heart attack requiring coronary artery bypass grafting, that person is two and a half times more likely to still be alive fifteen years down the road than someone who is unmarried. And when it comes to cancer, marriage can be more effective than chemotherapy. When researchers followed over 700,000 patients with several different types of cancer, they noticed that those who were married had between 12 and 33 percent higher chances of survival than their unmarried counterparts. That's higher than is usually found for the effects of chemotherapy.

Overall, the effects of marriage on longevity far surpass those commonly found for healthy eating or exercise. In one large sample, not being married meant even three times the risk of death for men, and a risk of 20 percent higher for women. The researchers who conducted the study called the effects "enormous"—and that's something coming from scientists, who are in general a cautious bunch when it comes to grandiose words. Yet the benefits of marriage are indeed enormous. Abundant research has now shown that from a health and longevity perspective, this is the most profitable relationship you can have. Marriage is not just better than exercise and diets; it's better than friendship, too—particularly if you are a man.

"It is a notorious fact that women everywhere are 'desperate to get married'" noted an article in the *Dallas Weekly Herald* back in 1882. Journalists these days may be more careful about making such statements, but in popular culture the image of a girl "desperate to get married" certainly lives on. However, men rather than women should be particularly keen on saying the vows. In study after study, it's the husbands who benefit the most from sporting a wedding ring, and who suffer exceedingly when their spouse dies. This so-called "widower effect" has been known for centuries—the 1657 mortality statistics for the city of London, England, listed such "griefe" as an official cause of death. There are plenty of stories of a spouse dying right after their partner passes away. When Ruth Kretschmer, a ninety-year-old afflicted with Alzheimer's disease, stopped breathing just before 10 a.m. one December morning, her husband of seventy-one years, Bob, passed away within fifteen minutes. They were both at their own house, lying in hospice beds just a few feet apart—while Ruth struggled with Alzheimer's disease, Bob had been fighting cancer. Once Bob heard that Ruth was gone, it seemed as if his body just gave up the struggle.

For new widows and widowers, the most dangerous period is the first week—the risk of dying from natural causes doubles for them. What's more, chances are that pets might suffer from a "widower effect," too. After our beloved cocker spaniel, Evita, passed away in August 2018, her longtime companion and our second dog, Roger, got diagnosed with an aggressive cancer just three weeks later. The veterinarian was not surprised. She told us such things happen often in her practice, to the despair of the pets' owners.

So what is it about marriage that gives those who go for it unprecedented longevity benefits? Maybe it's simply that the healthiest people get married in the first place, while the less strong-bodied ones remain spinsters and bachelors? Yet when studies control for pre-selection into marriage, the effects on health remain. Something else is obviously going on. Perhaps it's about economic factors—after all, the pooling of resources that happens with marriage is better for the wallet, which may translate into better health care access, better nutrition, and so on. But once again, financial well-being does not account for all the longevity perks of matrimony.

By now you may be wondering whether the key here is marriage as an institution, with ivory dresses, first dances, and white doves released into the sunset, or if maybe just living together—or "cohabiting," as scientists prefer to say—is good enough, too. It may be, it may not—it simply depends. A hefty pile of evidence suggests that it's all about commitment.

Voodoo Weddings and Synchronized Bodies

The Marché des Féticheurs, the world's largest outdoor voodoo market on the outskirts of Lome, Togo, smelled of dust and the sweetish, leathery scent of animal skins drying in the sun. The locals call this place "a pharmacy" and venture here to buy treatments for all ailments—from a porcupine quill for asthma to a mahogany seed for poor memory. As I walked among the stalls, clouds of rust-coloured soil rose up, settling slowly on everything around: dried crocodiles, chopped-off dogs' heads, birds with their eyes plucked out. Maciek, my better half, whom I had married many years previously in Poland, strolled beside me, bewilderment obvious on his face.

To the disappointment of the stall-keepers we decided against investing in animal skulls, but when one of the voodoo priests urged us inside his amulet shop, we followed him into the dusty interior. And when he offered to fortify our marriage vows with a few voodoo spells, we looked at each other, swallowed hard, and agreed. Couldn't hurt, right?

The ceremony was short and completely bewildering. The priest, who introduced himself as Germain, sang songs, rattled amulets, prayed to a giant clay statue of a voodoo god, and had us hold our hands and nod at certain intervals. Then he drank some liquid out of a jar with a dead snake inside, and rattled amulets some more. It all looked very serious.

I have to admit: after the voodoo ritual I felt even more committed to my dear husband than I had before. And no, it wasn't really about any worry that I might mess with some dark spirits by not being a perfectly devoted wife. It was more about deciding to honour our relationships within another culture, once again. To say yes in one more way. According to science, that voodoo ceremony might have prolonged my life.

A lot of research has found that simply living together as a couple is not as good for your physical well-being as is getting married. In a Finnish study published in 2015, those who cohabited without "putting a ring on it" had higher risk of heart attacks than did married people. For women, living out of wedlock was actually worse than being single—cohabitation meant 69 percent higher risk of a heart attack than being married, while those living on their own had that risk elevated only by 8 percent.

World-renowned marriage expert John Gottman, professor emeritus of psychology at the University of Washington, believes that it's the strength of commitment that is responsible for the health and longevity benefits of marriage. He believes that is why cohabitation may not offer the same gains. Gottman told me about a fascinating experiment in which holding hands reduced the activity of the amygdala in gay couples, but only if they considered themselves married (that was before same-sex marriage became legal in the US). "In any relationship that can create that sense of trust and commitment, people will get the benefits," Gottman told me. Researchers in general distinguish two types of cohabiting couples: those who intend to stay together "till death do us part," and those who don't. It's only the former who may reap the health benefits of a romantic relationship. So if you want to live long, it might be a good idea to adopt the viewpoint of Audrey Hepburn, who once said, "If I get married, I want to be very married."

That a loving marriage may give you oxytocin and dopamine boosts and calm down your HPA axis seems quite straightforward. But what if the marriage is bad? What if all you do is bicker all day? What if there is more serious abuse? The evidence here is divided. In some studies, all wives and husbands come out ahead of single people in terms of health, even with all the dysfunctional relationships thrown in the mix.

Some researchers argue that a less-than-perfect marriage may still have some advantages for physical fitness since signing up for the institution of matrimony may bring with itself a greater inclusion in society at large, a kind of embeddedness. Still, plenty of studies show that the quality of your marriage does matter—a lot. That's particularly true for women. For both spouses, low marital satisfaction has been linked to physiological processes that can lead to diabetes, elevated inflammation, poor response to viruses, bad arteries, and even bad teeth. Happily married women, meanwhile, are three times less likely to develop metabolic syndrome than are those stuck in a loveless relationship. And yes, love is key here. Two Chinese studies have found that arranged marriages don't bring the same levels of well-being as so-called "love marriages," no matter what conservative Asian parents may tell you. It appears that for a real commitment, your heart must be in it.

One of the reasons loving marriages work well for health is oxytocin. In one rather unpleasant experiment, a few dozen married
couples were invited into a lab, where researchers collected blood
samples for oxytocin and used small vacuum pumps to create blisters on the spouses' arms. Each of the couples was then asked to
discuss an important personal topic under surveillance by camera.
The conversations were subsequently ranked for hostility, humour,
support, and so on. Over the next twelve days, the couples came
repeatedly into the lab to have their blisters evaluated for speed of
healing. As you probably suspect, those who displayed the most positive behaviours during the discussion—such as humour, acceptance,
and self-disclosure—tended to have higher levels of oxytocin, and
their blisters healed the fastest, too.

The thing is that when you "tie the knot," you don't do it only
proverbially. You almost literally tie your physiology together as well.
Scientists call this "physiological linkage"—a situation in which the
bodily states of two people get synchronized. Romantic couples tend
to synchronize their blood pressure, cortisol levels, pulse, heart rate,
finger temperature, and electrical activity in the chest. One of the
reasons for such linkage, beyond the obvious—we both watch a scary
movie at the same time, so we are both scared—is the existence of
mimicry and mirror neurons (more on these in the next chapter).

Just like marriage, physiological linkage can be for better or for
worse. If your spouse has high levels of stress hormones in the blood
throughout the day, you are likely to have similar levels, too, whether
you are fighting or not. In general, partners who are more responsive to one another tend to have "healthier" profiles of stress hormones, which in turn keeps the immune system functioning well,
too. Being apart, meanwhile, may play havoc with sleep quality and
the functioning of the HPA axis—even if the separations are as short
as four to seven days. And it's not just the physiology of the couple
that suffers; their emotional connection tends to go downhill, too.

The most affected are those who already have a tendency to be anxious about their relationships to begin with. What helps in such situations, researchers have found, are long phone calls. Not a lot of short check-ins, mind you, but lengthy conversations. And not emails or text messages, either.

Divorce, on the other hand, spells trouble for your centenarian potential. Being divorced means about 30 percent higher risk of death—giving up on your spouse is comparable to giving up completely on eating fresh fruits and veggies (in one meta-analysis, zero servings of fruits and vegetables a day versus six meant 26 percent higher mortality risk). In case you were wondering: so far it hasn't been really investigated whether staying in a bad marriage is worse for your health than divorce. What we do know is that the effects of divorce are relatively independent of culture and quite similar across the planet, whether in the US, Scandinavia, Bangladesh, Brazil, or Lebanon. And no, Americans are not the most divorce-prone nation. That would be the inhabitants of the Maldives: the rate of divorce per year per thousand Americans is 2.9, while in the Maldives it's a whopping 10.97. It seems that honeymoon-like scenery is not enough to keep a marriage alive. Far more important are positivity, gratitude, and visiting amusement parks.

The Four Horsemen of the Apocalypse

She wore a flowing, lacy veil that pooled at her feet. He had a white bow tie and a slightly skittish expression. It's been eighty-six years since John and Ann Betar got immortalized in their black-and-white wedding photo. The year was 1932, the place: Harrison, New York, a small town northeast of Manhattan. John and Ann had eloped after just days of dating. She was seventeen. He, a Syrian refugee, was twenty-one. People said it wouldn't last—but it did. At the time of writing they were both well over a hundred and seemed enviably happy together. In photos, their smiles are wide and their eyes twinkle behind matching glasses.

Certainly for the Betars, named the "longest-married couple in America," good marriage did seem to pair with good health—as late as 2018 they were both still active and independent, even as centenarians. They lived on their own, cooking from scratch together and reading books. Their secret to a happy, long-lasting relationship? "We never hold grudges. Most arguments are about food," John said. To which Ann replied: "Yeah, like, 'You bought the wrong kind of cucumber!'" In a more serious moment, Ann admitted that the key to their success is respect for each other. "We are not arguing; we are listening. And we've always listened," she said.

The Betars may be on to something. In his decades-long research, John Gottman has shown over and over that skilful arguing is vital for marriage quality (and hence for health). In one of his more famous experiments, Gottman discovered that it was possible to predict whether a couple would stay married over the next fourteen years with 93 percent accuracy simply by observing for fifteen minutes how the husband and wife interacted while discussing a conflict-inducing topic (money, kids, chores). "We first look at the ratio of positive to negative emotions during that fifteen-minute conversation. In relationships that are stable and happy, that ratio of positive to negative averages five to one, whereas in relationships that are unstable it averages 0.8 to one—so it's quite a big difference," he told me.

The four things that really predict a demise of a relationship are criticism, defensiveness, contempt, and stonewalling, things that Gottman likes to call "the Four Horsemen of the Apocalypse," with the most powerful one being contempt. In good relationships, contempt is basically absent. How do you spot it? "It's saying things like, "You're so ridiculous, that's the kind of person you are, you're a slug," explains Gottman. Criticism, meanwhile, is stating your complaint as a defect in your partner's personality. "If I were to criticize my wife, I might say, 'You're so selfish, all you think is yourself! You don't care about me.' That's criticism. In a good relationship I might say, 'You know, I get lonely when you're on your cell phone doing your email when we're having dinner. I really would like it if you would turn off your cell phone.' Much more specific and clear, and not an attack on her personality," Gottman says.

The next in line is defensiveness—playing the victim, denying any responsibility for the marital problems. Last but not least, stonewalling—completely ignoring your partner. Maybe you turn on the TV during the fight or start texting on your phone. Don't do that, Gottman says. Instead, just like the Betars, listen, always listen. Focusing on the other person can help you stay calm during conflict and enable communication—two things that are key when you fight.

If you fight nasty, not only may your marriage not survive, but you might also get . . . fat. There was one experiment, published in 2016, that began very similarly to the one conducted by Gottman. The couples who volunteered for the study had to discuss a conflict topic for twenty minutes while their behaviours were recorded and then assessed by researchers for hostility, criticism, eye-rolling, etc. Yet the goal here was not to predict who would stay together for years to come—it was to investigate the inner workings of the couples' digestive systems.

After the marital squabbling session was over, the husbands and wives were served a fatty meal which totalled almost a thousand calories: they got eggs, turkey sausage, biscuits, and gravy. For the next seven hours, the volunteers remained at the lab while their bodily functions were repeatedly measured. Here is what was found: men and women who fought most unpleasantly and who also had a history of depression had lower resting energy expenditure, higher insulin, and higher peak triglyceride responses after the greasy meal. Their bodies were not dealing well with all that fat. The difference in energy intake from the food between the dirty fighters and those who were nicer to their spouses was 128 calories. Over a year, that could add up to almost eight pounds (3.6 kg) of extra weight. In other words: rolling eyes at your spouse could make you fat.

Are you an eye-roller? Does your partner stonewall you? If you are married or living together, yet it's not all roses and rainbows, the good news is that you can likely improve your relationship and still reap the health and longevity benefits of a romantic bond. And no, spraying OxyLuv up your partner's nose is not the only solution. Most people can be taught how to fight well, Gottman told me. When I asked him directly if he believed that most marriages could be saved from divorce, his answer was a resounding yes. He often advises couples who come to see him to turn toward their partner's attempt to connect emotionally and communicate affection and respect in a relationship. "Try to stay calm when you are disagreeing with your partner—that allows you to listen and communicate understanding," he says.

Other research shows that sharing good news with your loved one may be more important than commiserating about mishaps and problems—counting your blessings together boosts positive emotions and injects happy feelings into the relationship. Try to look for opportunities to update your significant other on the pleasant parts of your day. Maybe someone was nice to you in traffic or your boss complimented your work. Share it. It could bring you closer. Not only will your relationship be better off for it, but also your health—after all, the powerful linkages between your emotions and your health through your HPA axis, your vagus nerve, and your gut microbiota mean that a happy marriage can mean a long life.

One more science-tested way of injecting more positivity into your marriage is creating something psychologists call a "positivity portfolio." Make a list of things you love about your spouse, place happy photos of the two of you around the house, and listen to your special songs from time to time. Remember what brought you together in the first place. Express gratitude. Look out for moments when your partner does something nice and thank them for it.

John Malouff, cognitive scientist at the University of New England, Australia, recommends another relationship-boosting technique— and a fun one, too. He calls it an "excitement program." When he tried this intervention with dozens of couples over a period of four weeks, the quality of the relationships improved significantly. Here is what you do: instead of having your marriage on autopilot, try novel and challenging activities together. Play more. Go on adventures. Each week, try to think of something you haven't done before, something both of you may enjoy. Rock climbing? Ice skating? Dining in darkness?

There are several reasons why this works. Not only can routine and boredom be killers of romantic relationships (that's rather obvious), but research also shows that doing thrilling activities with someone you are attracted to fools your body on a physiological level. When we get a boost of adrenaline, we tend to misinterpret it as a thrill of sexual attraction—the kind of butterflies you get at the very beginning of a romantic relationship but which inevitably fade over time. Cross a suspension bridge with your other half and you may feel as if you've just met.

When I read Malouff's suggestions, it all sounded great, but hard to implement regularly when you have underage humans living with you (that is, kids). I could go canoeing with my husband or visit an amusement park once every few months, but doing it more often seemed overwhelming. Imagine the babysitting costs! When I raised this point with Malouff, he suggested that simpler things may also work well (on this book's website, there is a link Malouff sent me with some ideas).

Following his advice, my husband and I started weekly "home dates with a twist." Up until now we tended to spend evenings sitting on the couch, just chatting. Good, but not good enough. Now we try to do something different every week. One time we danced to our favourite songs from years ago. Another evening we did yoga together in our living room. Yet another we picked a "newlywed game" and quizzed each other on our favourite chocolate bars and most hated songs. And I was surprised to discover that there were still things I didn't know about my husband of eighteen years. Like the fact that the cartoon character I remind him of most is Lisa Simpson. Oh, well.

Whether you go skydiving together or simply learn not to roll your eyes at each other and to express gratitude, if you work on it, marriage may be potentially the most health-improving relationship to have. But good friendships are a close next. After all, even fruit flies have shorter lives if they don't have BFFs.

BFFs Make You Live Longer

One: "If one friend is bitten by a zombie, the other can't kill him."

Two: "If one friend gets superpowers, he will name the other one as his sidekick."

Three: "If one friend gets invited to go swimming at Bill Gates's house, he will take the other friend to accompany him."

Sheldon Cooper of *The Big Bang Theory* obviously took his friendships very seriously when writing the above clauses of the "Roommate Agreement" to be signed with his buddy, Leonard. Although most of us don't worry about the impact of potential zombie invasions on our social ties, we should all take a deeper look at our friendships. Our health and longevity may well depend on it.

Humans are not the only species to form friendships. Horses do that, monkeys do that, and so do giraffes, chimpanzees, spotted hyenas, donkeys, elephants, and even guppies. Male dolphins enjoy synchronous swimming with their mates, while horse "girlfriends" gently bite hard-to-reach spots on each other's necks to remove dead skin and untangle hair. Cows stand close to their friends and exchange licks. And with sociable animals, if you take their friends away, things go downhill. When such animals are isolated, their longevity suffers: lonely horses live shorter lives, and so do lonely fruit flies. Mice don't take well to seclusion, either. They get fat, develop type 2 diabetes, and even sleep poorly.

Similar things happen with humans. In Japan, older men who meet their friends less than a few times per year have 30 percent higher risk of dying than those who hang out with their mates at least once per month. That's a bigger disadvantage than going from eating six portions of fruits and vegetables a day to nothing (as you may remember, that increases mortality risk by "just" 26 percent). For women, these numbers were even more astounding: in this particular study, rarely meeting friends meant almost two and a half times the risk of a premature death. Even smoking comes up short in comparison (it elevates mortality risk by about 80 percent for smokers who puff more than ten cigarettes per day).

Although one study is probably not enough to claim that rarely meeting your friends is certainly worse for a woman than inhaling nicotine (which is really, really bad), it does signal the potential scale of the issue. And such effects are commonly found in research. When scientists studied elderly twins in Denmark, they also discovered that frequent contact with friends meant lower risk of dying— and again, the effects were particularly strong for women. The reason for this may lie in differences between male and female friendships. Psychologists say that for women friendships are "face-to-face," meaning that they are all about sharing emotions, while for men they are "side-by-side," so more about doing stuff together (like swimming in Bill Gates's pool). What's more, women in general tend to put more value on friendship and derive more meaning from it, and as we'll see in chapters 9 and 11, meaning in life is also important for health.

The impact of friendship on longevity is so large that in many studies it overshadows the impact of how often you meet with your relatives (not counting your spouse or a twin, if you have one). The reason for this, psychologists argue, may be that when we meet with our in-laws or aunts and uncles we sometimes do so simply out of obligation, which puts a shadow on any potential emotional benefits we may derive from the encounter.

Here is a thing, though. While identifying who is your spouse or your family member is easy (unless you live in a telenovela), how do you know who is your friend? Over three thousand years ago, the Vedas, a collection of religious texts written in ancient India, listed what a real friend should do, Sheldon Cooper–style: friends should provide food, protect one another's honour, and never abandon each other in times of need. In the twenty-first century, Western researchers find that people tend to define friends as those who offer us day-to-day assistance and as people with whom we share activities and secrets. Of course, in the digital era of Facebook and Snapchat, the way we see friendships is changing, and not necessarily for the better (more on that later).

There is no gold standard for how many friends are required for you to stay healthy and live long, but you certainly need a fairly large number of strong social connections whom you meet frequently. Scientists have invented plenty of different measures in their attempts to find an answer to "how much is enough." Generally, both the number of friends and how often you meet them seems to matter for health. In some studies, the minimum frequency is once every two weeks, while in others, the more often the better (at least once per week).

As for the number of friends, it seems more important to meet your specific needs than to strive for some gold standard of two, three, or four BFFs. Do you get invited to go out and do things with other people? Could you find someone to drive you places if you needed it? Do you have someone to help if you are sick in bed? Do you have a friend who will listen when you need to talk? While it may seem that a romantic partner may be enough to supply all this, plenty of research reveals that having both a significant other and friends is the best scenario. A Dutch study showed, for example, that each additional contact in your network with whom you have regular interactions, be it a spouse, a child, a sibling, a parent, a parent-in-law, a close friend, or a neighbour, lowers your risk of dying within the next five years by two percent. Family and friends can be substituted for one another to some extent, though—for example, the well-being of grandmothers who have good contact with their kids is comparable to that of childless old women surrounded by friends, while people who have fewer siblings and cousins tend to make up for such shortages by having more friends.

Yet all this doesn't mean that you should strive to collect as many friends as possible. University of Oxford anthropologist Robin Dunbar has famously calculated that humans can support only one to two special friends, about five intimate friends, and 150 "kind-of" friends. A special friend is basically your BFF. As for the five intimate friends, Dunbar told me that we should think about these people as our "shoulders to cry on" circle. "These are the people you go to for emotional support, social support, financial support, or when a crisis is happening, and it varies among people from about three to seven. We don't know why that varies, but that's the range. The average is five," Dunbar told me. This is supported by studies of hunter-gatherer tribes. Among the San of Botswana, for instance, women have on average 3.8 friends in their "hair-care" networks, meaning the groups of women who groom each other to pick out lice.

The 150 "kind-of" friends, meanwhile, are the people with whom we can support meaningful relationships. Dunbar has calculated that number based on the correlation between neocortex size and group size across primates—he basically checked how many "friends" each brain size can support. For humans, that works out to about 150, which is now known as "Dunbar's number." Our inner computers simply can't comfortably deal with more buddies.

It's not surprising, then, that the most common number of so-called "friends" on Facebook is between 150 and 250. But many psychologists warn that we should be careful with Facebook friendships. Two large studies published in 2017 and conducted on over a thousand people found that even though real-life friendships boosted self-reported health, Facebook ones did not. In yet another, high proportions of Facebook friends to offline ones meant higher levels of social isolation and loneliness.

The reason for these results may be the lack of deep emotional connection when we communicate over apps and websites. When pairs of friends were asked to talk either face-to-face or online, the degree of emotional bonding was the lowest among those who chatted over a messaging system. Other research reveals that hearing your mom's reassuring words on the phone causes a larger oxytocin release than does receiving similar support through a text message.

And although Facebook and its cousins can help some of us overcome loneliness (especially people who struggle with conditions like agoraphobia or physical disabilities), large societal trends suggest that our increasing reliance on online relationships is not helping us live happily ever after. Consider this: in the US between 2000 and 2015, the number of teenagers who went out with their friends almost every day plummeted 40 percent, while the rates of teen suicide went through the roof (it's been increasing on average by 6 percent a year since 2011). Heavy use of social media is often blamed as the likely cause of such changes. After all, young people who spend the most hours glued to their smartphones are most likely to have suicidal thoughts, and to suffer from depression and garden-variety unhappiness.

This may have something to do with social rejection, or what it's often called these days, FOMO—fear of missing out. Just think of what people post on Facebook, Instagram, and Snapchat: images of happiness, parties, fancy holidays, and delicious foods eaten with friends in hip restaurants. You see it, and if you are not there, you feel left out. As you may recall from previous chapters, even being excluded in *Cyberball,* a simple computer game, makes people feel lonely and activates neural networks that normally respond to physical pain. Although research on social media is only now picking up, we may soon see studies testing how our brains respond to FOMO experienced through Instagram or Snapchat. I bet that response will be at least as powerful as the response to shunning through *Cyberball*.

What's more, connecting online simply can't provide us with trust-enhancing physical warmth or offer the same boost of social neuro-peptides as does holding a friend's hand or getting a hug. Some of those working with digital communicators technology are beginning to realize these are serious drawbacks and are developing techno-logical remedies. Huggy Pajama, for instance, is a jacket you connect to the internet that can reproduce a hug remotely. One person embraces a doll that has embedded pressure-sensing circuits, while another can feel the touch through the compression and warmth re-created by the Huggy Pajama. A similar invention, HotHands, is based on personalized casts of your hand and that of your partner. When you talk using Skype or FaceTime, you place your palm onto the model hand, which causes the other person's model to warm up, too. Whether people who use HotHands or Huggy Pajamas really feel connected, and whether these tools can even partially replace the power of real, offline touch remains to be seen. I have to admit, I have my doubts.

Technology also likely won't solve another common relationship grievance created by smartphones and social media: phubbing. Even if you haven't heard the word yet, you have likely experienced the phenomenon: being ignored by someone who turns away from you to attend to their phone. The word comes from a mix of "snub-bing" and "phone," and already has sub-varieties, such as "p-phub-bing" ("partner"+"phubbing"). We've all seen it in practice. A family at a restaurant table, all checking their phones instead of talking. A parent at a playground cold-shouldering a whiny toddler to post an Instagram photo. A friend picking up a phone mid-conversation to reply to a text that's just arrived.

I've been guilty of phubbing myself on more occasions than I'd like to admit (women, in general, phubb more often than men do).

It may appear to be just a simple annoyance, but in reality phubbing is a type of ostracism, with all its relationship- and health-damaging consequences. Research that's just beginning to emerge shows that phubbing makes the offline conversation appear somehow less satisfying to us, the harmful effects spilling over to taint our perception of the whole relationship with the phubber or phubbee. In other words: the more you text and check your Instagram feed, the lower your partner will rate your relationship—and so will you.

If phubbing, smartphone addiction, and social media damage our perception of the value of our relationships, it follows that they may harm our health and even shorten our lives (and not just because some smartphones explode). To stave off heart disease, diabetes, and even cancer, what you need are high-quality friendships that you nurture offline, while your phone is far, far, away.

BFFs and KOFs

When my daughter was three years old, all she needed to find a new BFF was about ninety seconds on the playground. If only things were that easy for adults. In a 2012 *New York Times* article that went viral, Alex Williams describes the hardships of making friends if you are over thirty: "Schedules compress, priorities change and people often become pickier in what they want in their friends. No matter how many friends you make, a sense of fatalism can creep in: the period for making B.F.F.'s, the way you did in your teens or early 20s, is pretty much over. It's time to resign yourself to situational friends: K.O.F.'s (kind of friends)—for now."

Williams illustrates his essay with a personal story, which starts, "It was like one of those magical blind-date scenes out of a Hollywood rom-com, without the 'rom.'" He met Brian, a screenwriter, through work, and over dinner discovered an instant "friend chemistry." The story of Alex and Brian does not end well, though. With busy schedules in the way, they've only managed to meet four times in as many years, and the budding friendship never blossomed.

Yet research does confirm that this kind of instant friend chemistry indeed exists. We certainly form first impressions fast. Within a hundred milliseconds of meeting a new person—that's around the duration of an average eye blink—we already judge how likable or trustworthy the other one is, and we stick to that judgement later on. Young women and people with open, conscientious personalities are more likely to enjoy such immediate connections.

C. S. Lewis may have been on to something when he wrote that "Friendship is born at that moment when one person says to another: 'What! You, too? Thought I was the only one.'" Similarity certainly aids in becoming friends—and that applies even to non-human apes. In zoos, chimpanzees spend the most time with those fellow cage-mates with whom they share certain personality characteristics, like boldness or sociabiltity. This suggests that our penchant for the "two peas in a pod" scenario may have deep evolutionary roots. What's more, we choose our friends based on their genes. Yes, really. Friends resemble each other on a genotypic level far above what you might expect from chance or from population stratification due to geography or social divides. The genes we are particularly after are those related to dopamine, such as *DRD2*.

It doesn't mean, however, that if you are looking for a BFF you should fixate on finding your own twin. In reality we become friends with people who are similar enough but share something else with us that might be even more important than personality or age: geography. Police trainees, for example, are more likely to become buddies with other trainees whose last names start with the same letter. The reason? Alphabetized seating in police academy classrooms. In a similar fashion, the layout of your house may matter, too. Among university students, those who live in apartments without ensuite bathrooms tend to have stronger interpersonal bonds with their roommates.

Here is a tip, then: if you want to make friends in the office, try to get a desk in a high-traffic area. Close to the kitchen, perhaps? That also raises the question of how McMansion-style houses affect the relationship quality of the people that inhabit them. If everyone has their own bathroom, their own TV, and so on, and the spaces inside are so vast that you rarely cross paths with your fellow family members, are you missing out on a close bond? Can your health suffer because of that? Going even further—could McMansions shorten lifespans? As you may have guessed, so far there is no research to check this out—I have an inkling, though, that there may very well be a connection between poor health and overly large houses.

Yet even if you are geographically challenged where friendships are concerned—say your office desk is in the building's Siberia, or you live off-grid in the literal Siberia—there are ways to strengthen bonds with people you already know. First, give out your secrets. Studies show that self-disclosure brings people closer together. You don't really like your job? Your mother-in-law gets on your nerves? Share it with your favourite acquaintance, and she may well become a friend. Second is a somewhat less obvious strategy: let the other person do you a favour to harness a psychological phenomenon known as the "Ben Franklin Effect," inspired by the founding father's quote: "He that has once done you a kindness will be more ready to do you another than he whom you yourself have obliged." It may seem counterintuitive, but according to this theory, people feel so good about helping others that they start liking those they've helped more—possibly because subconsciously we want to reconcile our actions with our thoughts: "I'm helping this guy, so it must mean he is nice, right? Otherwise, why would I be doing this?"

Last but not least—commit more time to your friendships. Set up regular "dates" with your friends, or even simply pick up a phone and call them. Obvious? Maybe, but think how much time we spend obsessing about weight loss, exercise routines, pesticides in food, etc. Considering the importance of friendships to our health and longevity, we should spend more time on them each day than we spend thinking about nutrition.

What if you are an introvert, though? If every additional friend prolongs our lives, do introverts live shorter ones? Unfortunately, so it seems. In several studies, highly extroverted people tended to outlive the rest. Among the elderly of Chicago, for instance, a high level of extraversion meant a 21 percent lower risk of death, and similar findings came from Japan and Sweden. The good news here is that personality is not set in stone, and even if you are very introverted there are things you can do to mitigate potential impacts on your centenarian potential (more on this in chapter 9). Besides, in one of his studies, Robin Dunbar has found that even though extroverts tend to have more friends, the quality of their relationships isn't necessarily any better than that of introverts. He told me that what's important is to work with whatever seems best for you: "you may choose to spread your emotional capital thickly among a few people or thinly among many people." So the tip here would be: if you are an introvert, make sure to take particularly good care of your close relationships—and remember to meet with your friends regularly.

⧗

If you can do just one single thing for your health and longevity, that thing should be finding a great partner and committing to the relationship. Marriage, and in particular a happy one, can stave off cancer, diabetes, heart disease, the flu—the list goes on. Not only does it calm our stress response and the HPA axis, it can also boost the release of health-relevant social hormones. The effects are so large that if a twenty-a-day smoker, instead of ditching the cigarette habit, found lasting love, health-wise they might still come out on zero: their mortality risk might just be the same as if they didn't smoke at all (of course, the best would be to not smoke and have love).

And then there is friendship—the close second when it comes to boosting your centenarian potential. Yet we sabotage such relationships by phubbing and by running away from in-person interaction for the deceptive ease of Facebook connections. But Facebook friendships don't translate into better health. For most of us, they don't bring higher well-being, either. And yes, we are busy. But often we could choose to invest our time in different ways. Do you really need that house renovation? Do you have to sign your kid up for five extracurricular activities? Take some time to consider how you're spending your time, attention, and energy—and perhaps invest it in some of the relationships around you instead.

The problem is that although marriage and friendships are great at keeping our minds and bodies in shape, they are hard work—of a type whose effects are hard to measure (no "grams of companionship" to count per day). It's so much easier to try to fix your health by changing your exercise routine or by trying a new fad diet. Nutrition and fitness are quantifiable and often come with easy instructions. To make a watercress smoothie, place a bunch of watercress in a blender. Add one tablespoon of chia seeds and two cups of soy milk, and mix. That's easy to follow. If you do twenty minutes of strength training on Monday and walk ten thousand steps on Tuesday you know you are doing well in terms of exercise. But how do you judge the quality of a marriage? How do you know if your friendships are strong enough? We, the people of the twenty-first century, like easy prescriptions and instant gratification. With relationships, these things are hard to get.

About 90 percent of Americans will marry at least once in their lifetimes, yet many take this social bond for granted. Consider how much time some of us commit to training for marathons or similar sporting events. Do you know anyone who, every day, allocates the same amount of effort to improving his or her romantic relationship—excluding newlyweds, that is? From a longevity perspective, that's not a good thing. We should spend at least as much time reading about marriage-improving strategies as we do about diets and fitness. If time is limited, it's better to skip a gym session than a date night.

The good news is that science has discovered quite a few strategies for improving our relationships all in one go. You can boost your empathy, work on your attachment style, and engage in something psychologists call "social grooming." What's more, some of these strategies are actually quite quantifiable and almost as easy to do as making a watercress smoothie (and potentially more pleasant). Even line dancing, it appears, can prolong your life.

A FEW SUGGESTIONS TO BOOST YOUR LONGEVITY

Prioritize your romantic relationship and really commit to it. Read books and articles on how to be a better partner. Avoid the Four Horsemen of the Apocalypse: contempt, criticism, stonewalling, and defensiveness. Talk with your spouse often about good things that happen in your daily life. Try new, exciting things together and have fun (rollercoasters and balloon rides are great). Invest in friendships. Spend more time together, disclose your secrets, and ask for favours. Stop phubbing your close ones—put your phone away and cut down on social media.

7

CHAMELEONS LIVE LONG

Empathy, Attachment, and Social Grooming

BACK IN THE 1960s, some people called the University of Wisconsin at Madison primate lab at 600 North Park Street the "Goon Park"—and not just because of the address—and the scientist who worked there, Harry Harlow, eccentric or even pure crazy. Yet no matter how odd the research done at Goon Park appeared at the time, it has changed the way we now see love and attachment—both between monkeys and between humans.

Harry Harlow was a brilliant man obsessed with fame, an alcoholic, and a workaholic whose experiments at the primate lab caused uproar among animal activists. Take the isolation studies he conducted on baby rhesus macaques, little creatures with round eyes and big ears. To study what would happen to monkeys deprived of social contact in early life, Harlow designed something he called "the pit of despair." It was a cage shaped like an inverted pyramid, wide at the top and narrow at the bottom, its roof made of wire mesh. A monkey would be placed inside, all alone. For the first two or three days it would try to flee, scrambling up the slippery sides to the top, where a mesh roof prevented its escape. Then it would give up. "Most subjects typically assume a hunched position in a corner of the bottom of the apparatus. One might presume at this point that they find their situation hopeless," Harlow wrote. Even a few days were enough to break a monkey. It would sit motionless at the bottom of the cage, staring blankly, head slumped. When these monkeys were returned to their families, they were withdrawn and unable to reconnect.

Not all Harlow's experiments were as horrific as these ones. You might have heard, for example, about his studies involving terry-cloth surrogate mothers. Baby macaques would be placed in a cage with two makeshift "mothers" to choose from. One would be made out of wire, perfect for climbing but with no soft edges to hug. The other would have a smiling face and a round body covered in sponge rubber and cotton terry cloth, heated by a light bulb. In some cases it was the soft mother that held a bottle of milk; in others, the metal one. No matter, though, which surrogate had the food, little monkeys invariably preferred the cloth mothers—they would cuddle up to them for hours and run to them when scared. When the surrogates needed to be taken out of the cages for cleaning, the baby monkeys bawled inconsolably. Physical warmth and simple touch, it seemed, were everything when it came to parenting primates.

These experiments, though less stomach-turning than the ones involving the "pit of despair," unfortunately also didn't have a happy ending. As they reached adulthood, macaques raised from infancy by sponge stand-in mothers started showing worrisome characteristics: they were shy and withdrawn, unsure how to behave around other monkeys. When they became mothers themselves, their parenting skills were pretty poor, too. Some were indifferent toward their babies, not nursing them. Others were outright abusive, biting and injuring their own offspring.

Over the years, the Goon Park experiments on love and sociality formed the basis of research on human attachment—the science of how early experiences with our caregivers shape us for life and determine our abilities to forge meaningful relationships with others. Just as Harlow's monkeys would become attached to their terry-cloth mothers, human infants get attached to their mothers, too—for better or for worse. How the relationship is going can be tested quite early on. If a mother leaves a twelve-month-old baby alone in a room with a stranger for a mere three minutes, after which the mother returns and the stranger exits, you can get an idea of how the infant is attached to the mother.

This procedure, known as the "Strange Situation," in its proper form includes a few more steps, such as leaving the baby completely on their own for a couple of minutes. Its basic simplicity, however, made it widely popular among researchers (and if you have a baby between twelve and eighteen months old you can try it at home, too). If the little one is distressed when the mother leaves the room yet happy on reunion, using her as a safe base to explore the surroundings, they are likely securely attached. If they are upset by being left with a stranger yet also upset with the mother when she returns, they are probably insecurely attached in a way that's considered "anxious." And if the mother's comings and goings don't seem to affect the baby at all, the assumption is that they are attached in an insecure-avoidant way. Any parent should want their child to be securely attached, but the reality is that only 65 percent of American babies are that way. In the UK, 75 percent are securely attached, while in China that number is just 50 percent.

Decades of research show that the consequences of insecure attachment in both its forms can be pretty dire, predicting depression, anxiety, and low self-esteem later in childhood. On the other hand, securely attached babies grow up to be more empathic, helpful preschoolers who are surrounded by friends. As preteens, they are more popular and socially competent.

Yet attachment is not just about babies—it can also be measured in adults. Do you know someone who is always on the lookout for the ways others may hurt their feelings? Who constantly worries what people think about them? Who gets easily offended and exaggerates emotions? What about someone who is dismissive and afraid of commitment and intimacy? People like that are avoid-antly attached—just like the babies who don't cry when their mom leaves them with a stranger. Those of us who are securely attached, meanwhile, tend to see the world as a generally safe place where other people can be counted on for help and support. The differ-ences between securely and insecurely attached people can be seen not just in their behaviours, but in their brains, too. Functional magnetic resonance imaging studies show that when people with avoidant attachment style meet their friends, the reward circuits in their brains don't light up as strongly as they do in adults who are securely attached.

There are plenty of indications that your attachment style truly matters for your health and longevity—for one, it can affect your physical well-being directly. For instance, adults with more attach-ment anxiety deal less well with a virus that can cause mononucleo-sis. Compared to securely attached people, those who are anxiously attached have more strokes and heart attacks, higher blood pres-sure, and more ulcers. They also suffer more often from medically unexplained musculoskeletal pain. To avoidantly attached people—those who agree with statements such as, "I find it difficult to allow myself to depend on romantic partners"—even a simple pinprick to the fingertip can feel particularly painful, much more so than to the happily attached people of the world.

Once again, the underlying cause for the links between attach-ment style and physical health appears to be the stress response and the functioning of the HPA axis. When insecurely attached people experience stress, their HPA axis becomes highly activated—it quickly dumps large quantities of cortisol into the body, which then takes a long time to return to baseline. Cortisol, in turn, can alter the work-ings of the immune system. In one study, people with high attach-ment anxiety had 22 percent fewer CD3+CD8+ cytotoxic T cells than those with lower attachment anxiety. These T cells are vital for the immune response since they kill pathogen-infected cells, and their reduced number is an indication of aging in the immune system. In other words, you could say that people who are anxiously attached have the worn-out immune systems of the elderly. And if that's not enough, insecure attachment can also mean poor self-control with food—it may be linked to eating disorders, and binge eating in particular. So if you ever find yourself in front of the fridge at midnight, consider that your attachment style may be to blame.

To make things worse, commitment-phobes tend to have higher fasting blood glucose levels, which is a warning sign for diabetes. This may have an evolutionary explanation. Blood glucose is the basic fuel of the body, and of the brain in particular. If you are alone on the savanna, you need to deal with threats on your own. Since there is no one else to warn you of predators, you have to be constantly ready for danger. Your brain and body need easily accessible metabolic resources to help with quick decision making—and so your blood glucose stays up.

Besides directly affecting your HPA axis or your blood glucose, your attachment style can also influence your centenarian potential indirectly by changing the quality of your relationships. People who are securely attached are happier with their friendships, fight less with their loved ones, and are less likely to end up divorced. On the flip side, insecurely attached people are not only less satisfied with their romantic partners, but with their kids as well. And even if they have as many friends as others do, they are often quite negative about the support they are getting. That, of course, is also a longevity wrecker.

Now, here is the big question: are you securely or insecurely attached? With babies the test may be fairly easy, but how do you assess attachment in adults? After all, I bet you don't cry when left for a few minutes alone with a stranger. To evaluate adult attachment, psychologists use several carefully designed questionnaires, in which they make you score statements such as, "I feel like I have someone to rely on," "I feel I can trust the people who are close to me," and "I feel a strong need to be unconditionally loved right now," with the last one being a sign of anxious attachment.

In general, about 55 to 65 percent of adults are securely attached, 22 to 30 percent are avoidant, and 15 to 20 percent are anxious in their attachment style. The bad news for both love and longevity, though, is that insecurity in attachment is on the rise. A large meta-analysis of studies of college students revealed that whereas in 1988 close to 50 percent of American youth were securely attached, by 2011 that number had dropped to 41 percent. The scientists behind the meta-analysis point out that smartphones and internet may be to blame for our "increased disconnection in an age of increased connection."

Wait a second, you may say, phones and internet? Isn't attachment all about the mother who was not involved enough, didn't breastfeed you, didn't babywear you, and didn't co-sleep with you? The answer is both yes and no. For an infant to be securely attached, you do need a caring, affectionate parent. The recipe is as follows (more or less, of course): take a sensitive, loving parent who responds to the baby's basic needs, and the little one will grow up believing that the world is a safe place and that people can be generally trusted. Simple in theory, harder in practice, if you consider attachment statistics. Parents who are inconsistent in how they respond to their children— lovingly one time, coldly or angrily another—tend to have anxiously attached children, while those who are often emotionally unavailable to their kids end up with mini commitment-phobes.

Yet although it may be tempting to blame your mom for your imperfect romantic life, your cardiovascular health, or your binge sessions in front of the fridge, how you were parented early in your life is not a sentence when it comes to attachment style. Many psychologists argue that adult attachment is flexible and can't be fully attributed to how you were parented. This is good news. Simply knowing that even if your mom's caregiving style wasn't Instagram-perfect you are not doomed to insecure attachment for lifetime—and hence busted health—can empower you to change the way things are. How to do it? The best solution is psychotherapy (sorry, no easy fixes here). Luckily, though, you don't necessarily need to spend years on a psychotherapist's couch and pay a gazillion dollars in fees. As little as six weeks of intensive therapy can boost security of attachment— and, hopefully, your health.

What's more, an additional side effect of enhanced attachment security can be higher empathy—another vital ingredient of a robust social life. If you want to live happily to a hundred, empathy is something you should certainly put on your self-improvement agenda, even if it means skipping a few trips to the gym or saying no to broccoli-cooking classes.

Laughter Epidemics, Phubbing, and the Empathy Crisis

On January 30, 1962, in the small village of Kashasha in northern Tanganyika (now Tanzania), something strange started happening at a local school. At first it was innocent enough: three of the local girls started laughing—and couldn't stop. But then things got considerably weirder: the incontrollable laughter went on spreading among the teenage students. For some, the laughing episode lasted a few hours. For others, it went on as long as sixteen days. By March 18, well over half the girls at the Kashasha school were affected and the school was temporarily closed down. Yet even that wasn't the end of the story. The laughter epidemic continued to widen its range, jumping from village to village. In total, about a thousand people ended up with the giggle-bug, girls and boys, students and adults alike, and fourteen schools were forced to shut their doors.

It was hardly a laughing matter. People were scared. Some believed that the event was caused by atmospheric pollution from an atomic bomb (that, of course, wasn't true). Others speculated that the local maize flour might have been poisoned. Doctors were called, blood was drawn and shoved under microscopes, lumbar punctures were performed, but no toxins, bacteria, or viruses were found. In fact, nothing was found. The people affected by the laughter epidemic were most likely perfectly healthy. Today, psychologists suspect that the Tanganyika laughter epidemic was caused by mass hysteria, and that it had something to do with mood transmission—an essential part of empathy.

Have you ever noticed that if someone beside you yawns, it's hard to resist doing the same? Even just reading about yawning may be causing you to stretch your mouth to inhale deeply right this very moment. Small epidemics of yawning, which can be observed anywhere from the metro to university classrooms, rely on similar mechanisms to that infamous Tanganyika outbreak of laughter. And the more empathic someone is, the more susceptible they are to the yawning contagion. For that reason, if you had a classroom full of psychopaths—admittedly a daunting prospect—the yawning would not spread.

Frans de Waal, a renowned Dutch primatologist, believes that mood contagion evolved so that primates such as our ancestors could coordinate their behaviour, a crucial thing for a species that travels in groups. If it's feeding time, we'd better all be eating. If it's walking time, we'd better all start going. Yet empathy is about far more than just simple mood transmission. It's also about adopting other people's perspectives, understanding their motivations, and being sensitive to their emotions. As Roman Krznaric, the author of *Empathy: Why It Matters, and How to Get It* cleverly puts it, empathy is about looking outward instead of inward.

Yet just like secure attachment, empathy may also be in crisis these days. A meta-analysis of studies done on over thirteen thousand American students showed that between 1979 and 2009, empathic concern for others nose-dived by 48 percent. Now consider that 2009 was still the early days for smartphones—the word "phubbing" hadn't even been invented yet. In one of his speeches, former president Barack Obama noted that "we live in a culture that discourages empathy." He blamed the looming empathy crisis on the selfish impulses promoted by our culture: to be entertained, famous, thin, and rich. Obama was right to point his finger at the pursuit of riches—studies confirm that those who are financially very well off tend to score low on empathy. He was also right that cultures are not created equal when it comes to "looking outward," although the US does not come out particularly badly in the rankings. In research conducted at Michigan State University, the US ranked seventh from the top among sixty-three countries, while Canada was twelfth and UK was forty-seventh. Ecuador proved to be the world's most empathic nation. At the very end of the list was Lithuania, while my native Poland scored fourth from the bottom.

Yet, to state the obvious, it's not just countries that differ in their levels of empathy—individual people do so, too. What's less obvious is that there are patterns to these differences. In general, women tend to be more empathic than men: over 66 percent of the time it will be the woman who will score higher on empathy. This difference is already apparent in toddlerhood, with two-year-old girls showing more concern for people in distress than do boys of the same age. De Waal argues that we've evolved this way: the empathy of the mother was more vital to the baby's survival than the empathy of the father—whether she was quick to nurse in response to hunger, for instance. So the infants of the most empathic mothers were the most likely to survive and carry on the genes.

Male fetuses are exposed to higher levels of testosterone during pregnancy, with effects on the brain. If a pregnant woman undergoes amniocentesis during the second trimester of pregnancy and the levels of testosterone in the amniotic fluid are measured, you can have quite a good shot at guessing how empathic her kid will be at school age. In a study of six- to eight-year-olds that followed such a procedure, the most "outward looking" kids were the ones who were exposed to the lowest levels of testosterone in their mother's bodies. Which is another good reason for not smoking while pregnant, since nicotine raises testosterone levels in the fetus. The testosterone-empathy connection is also a perfect excuse for expecting mothers to put their feet up more often—just like nicotine, maternal cortisol may hike up fetal testosterone (note to future moms: now you can claim that that relaxing maternity massage is totally for the baby).

In the testosterone study, the children were evaluated with a test commonly used to asses empathy called "Reading the Mind in the Eyes." If you want to check your own empathy levels, it's a fun way to do so: your task is to look at photos of human eyes and guess what emotion the portrayed person is experiencing (there are links to the test on this book's website). Another tool to assess your empathy is also available there—"Empathy Quotient," which is a more standard survey-type test.

Why does that all matter for your longevity? Just like its relative, attachment, empathy plays a vital role in health by affecting our relationships. Take a teenager, measure their empathy levels, and you will be able to predict how socially well-integrated they will be two decades later as a thirty-something. Empathy also has a potent anti-loneliness effect. No matter your age, the more empathic you are, the less likely you are to feel all alone in the world. For marriage, too, high empathy means better quality, in a roundabout way adding years to our lifespans. Several studies have uncovered that higher empathy in the spouses predicts more relationship satisfaction, with the husband's "outward looking" skills being more vital than the wife's.

This may all seem daunting if you suspect your empathy levels may not be of Dalai Lama quality. What if you are a Lithuanian man whose overly stressed mother chain smoked in pregnancy? Are you doomed? The good news is that empathy can be increased, although it may require some effort.

Empathy 101

On a hot, stuffy day in London, UK, in a bright, white-walled class-room of the Ashburnham Primary School, two dozen nine- and ten-year-olds sat in a circle around a green blanket. There, in the middle of that woven stage, lay a ten-month-old baby, clad in a onesie with "Roots of Empathy" written across the tummy. Her name was Evelyn, and today she was the star. Everyone's eyes followed her as she strained to reach a pink plush clam that had rolled away. Libby, Evelyn's mom, helped her get the toy and started playing with it, making it squeak repeatedly. At first, Evelyn was curious, but she soon got upset. She whimpered in frustration. "Too much, baby?" Libby asked.

Christine Zanabi, an empathy instructor, turned to the big children: "Did you notice what the mom said?" A girl with long, strawberry-blond hair replied: "She said, 'too much.'" The instructor nodded: "So mom is really tuned in to how the baby is feeling, 'It's a bit too much, it's too exciting.' We saw the mom help the baby regulate her feelings." The instructor paused, then continued. "When you are feeling upset, how do you regulate yourself? What to do you do to feel a little bit calmer?" Hands shot up, and a girl was chosen to reply, "To calm myself, I draw." Then another: "I sing." Christine suggested that singing may soothe the baby too, so the students picked up a tune: "Hush little baby, don't say a word . . ." Evelyn watched them intently and stopped crying. "What's happened when you were singing?" Christine asked. An answer came: "She went much more quiet." The instructor then pointed out to the children that they sang the song more softly than they usually do, subcon-sciously tuning in to the baby's needs. She asked them to recall the times in their lives when they experienced frustration, the way Evelyn did when playing with the toy. Once again, many hands rose.

What I witnessed that day in London was part of a program called "Roots of Empathy" run by a Canadian non-profit with the same name. The idea is to teach children emotional literacy so that they become more sensitive and socially integrated human beings. The babies in the program are the "teachers"—by observing their development over the course of several months, by labelling their feelings and comparing them to what they experience in their own lives, the students, ages five to thirteen, learn to be more empathic. As a result, classroom bullying goes down while pro-social behaviours go up. According to the research done on the program, the results last for at least a year after the intervention.

Many other studies confirm that training empathy does indeed work. It works for children, resident physicians, and sex offenders. The curricula differ, but they usually offer a mixture of such approaches as learning to decode facial expressions, improving listening skills, and mastering how to take the perspective of another person. Some actors can be a good example of how investing a lot of effort into empathy can pay off. Take Nicolas Cage. For his role of a Vietnam vet in *Birdy*, Cage had a few teeth pulled out, without anaesthesia, and kept his face wrapped in bandages for weeks. "When I took the bandages off, my skin was all infected because of acne and ingrowing hairs," he told the *Telegraph*. To play a Holocaust survivor in *The Pianist*, Adrien Brody starved himself to drop thirty pounds, practised piano for four hours a day, and, as if that wasn't enough, he gave up his apartment, sold his car and moved to Europe with nothing but two bags and a keyboard. All so that he would feel as lost as his character did.

Cage's and Brody's so-called "method acting" is certainly going a bit far when it comes to practising empathy, but Roman Krznaric vouches that similar efforts on an everyday scale can indeed improve our "outward looking"—and so, presumably, our health. Krznaric argues that empathy, like every other skill, takes practice, and you should make a conscious decision to work on it. To do so, you should develop curiosity about others and try seeing the world through their eyes, letting go of preconceived ideas. How does life look to your dark-skinned waiter at an Indian restaurant? Where do you think your taxi driver goes after she is off duty? Does she seem tired to you? Happy? What is your kid really feeling when he is whining before dinner?

While these are good starting points, Krznaric encourages you to go even further than simply engaging in mental exercises—he recommends "experiential adventures," trying out other people's lives yourself, even if you can only dip your toes into other existences. You could take part in a charity-organized fundraiser where you sleep on the streets with homeless people. You could fast for Ramadan with your Muslim friends or go to mass with your Catholic ones. You could trade jobs with someone for a day or try dining in the dark to empathize with blind people (restaurants in many cities now offer such experiences). On a smaller scale, certain books and movies can also help us practise empathy—if you've ever cried in a cinema or while reading a novel you probably know what I mean. Krznaric has developed what he calls an "online empathy library" with reviews and charts of the most empathy-inspiring books and films.

Even the most empathy-resistant testosterone-loaded Lithuanian man can be taught to be very "outward looking." In one experiment, men scored much worse than women on understanding emotion until the researchers offered to pay them for their effort, proportionally to their performance. The monetary incentive was enough to wipe out any differences in empathy between the male and female participants (if you are female and married, and you are now considering whether paying your husband to listen better would be a good idea, I can only say—try it, who knows, it might well work).

What does hurt empathy, though, is, ironically, pain medication. In case you are prone to taking acetaminophen pills such as Tylenol, consider that a 2016 study showed that it can reduce empathic concern for other people's aches and throbs. So if your partner's headache or sore back doesn't seem like such a big deal to you, the reason may be the pill you've recently taken for your own pains. What could help you reconnect in such a situation, other than waiting for the acetaminophen to flush out of your system, would be for you to try dancing together or singing a song, the more synchronously the better. And yes, I'm serious. So-called "social grooming" such as synchronous dancing, choir singing, or synchronized sports not only bonds people but also improves health.

Why Disco Dancing and Choir Singing Are Good for Health

At a conference on the archaeology of music held in Reading, UK, Robin Dunbar, the Oxford anthropologist whom I've interviewed about our social brains, had a flash of insight while engaged in traditional Zulu dancing. It was early evening, and most of the serious talks were over, when an unusual exercise was suggested: the gathered academics were to walk around in an African dance, blowing on pieces of plastic tubing cut to different sizes. "Just wait and see what happens," the instructor said. And so walk they did, in a group of about twenty, and blow they did, creating a rather unpleasant ruckus. Yet after about five minutes the sounds and movements changed—without particular effort, the scientists became synchronized, playing music in consistent tune with each other. "It really was extraordinary; you could feel this uplift from doing it," Dunbar told me, adding that he now suspects that the feeling of exhilaration was created by the release of endorphins.

In the years since the Zulu dance, Dunbar has extensively researched synchrony and the astounding effects it has on our body. In one of his experiments, simple disco dancing was enough to bring about social closeness and improve physiological health. A few dozen people were asked to learn four basic dance routines from a video. This part of the experiment must have been quite fun, the volunteers mastering such classic moves as "driving" (one hand is extended as if resting on top of a steering wheel, crossing from left to right and back, while the other hand hangs relaxed along the body) or the "swimming move" (knees bending rhythmically, arms alternating from side to side as if doing the front crawl).

Afterward, the participants were divided into groups of four. Everyone was given headphones through which music started flowing and the disco began. In some of the groups, volunteers heard the same music and were instructed to do exactly the same moves, causing them to dance synchronously, while in other groups people jigged in total chaos—everybody to their own, different tune. Once the admittedly weird disco was over, research assistants pulled blood pressure–measuring monitors onto the arms of each dancer, asking them to indicate when the discomfort of the inflating cuff became uncomfortable. In reality the scientists were not interested in the cardiac health of the volunteers, but rather in their pain thresholds. And they got some interesting findings: those dancers who boogied in sync could stand the monitor's cuff clamping over their arms much more tightly than did those who didn't engage in synchrony. What's more, they also claimed to be feeling friendlier with the other volunteers, or in science-speak, "socially closer."

Many other studies conducted by Dunbar and his colleagues have found similar effects of doing things in synchrony. Singing in a choir causes release of endorphins, natural painkillers, and makes people feel more included and more connected to others. Rowing in a group, as compared to rowing alone, makes pain more bearable. Singing and dancing synchronously incites people to donate money and increases trust. Even tapping your fingers in rhythm with a partner works, promoting warm feelings of togetherness. Unfortunately, it doesn't mean you can eat all the fast food in the world as long as you tap your fingers in sync with someone a few times a day (I can only imagine tables full of finger-tapping customers at McDonald's). Synchrony increases feelings of closeness, but obviously doesn't have the same health-boosting powers as being surrounded by trusted friends.

Dunbar told me that singing and dancing, and in particular of the synchronous kind, likely plays such an important role in our social lives for evolutionary reasons. In order to bond and keep the group together, non-human primates groom each other. I groom you, you groom me, then I go on to groom ape X and you to ape Y, and so on. Picking fleas out of another's fur takes a lot of time, though, and Dunbar calculated that it sets an upper limit on the size of a group that can be bonded at about fifty individuals. That's not much.

As you may recall, Dunbar's number of how many close friends a human can have stands at around 150—three times the flea-picking maximum. So what has likely happened is that we've come up with ways to "groom" several people at once—using our voices or the movements of our bodies instead of our fingers. Just like classic grooming—I rub you, you rub me—singing and dancing release social neurohormones, such as endorphins and oxytocin, into the body, which helped our ancestors bond. This may also in part explain why ritualized dancing and singing is so widespread across cultures, from the tribes of Pacific islands to the Inuit of the North, and the peculiar appeal of flash mobs at the turn of the twenty-first century.

When we dance or sing in synchrony, as opposed to just jigging or humming in dissonance, the endorphin kick can double. "We really don't know why that might be the case; it's a big puzzle," Dunbar told me. He suspects, however, that the endorphin boost of synchrony may be due to the workings of our so-called mirror neurons. These are the brain cells that fire when we observe others acting and simulate the behaviour in our own neural system.

We humans are so sensitive to synchrony that even fourteen-month-old babies prefer a teddy bear with which they rock in their seat in synchrony to another that moves at a different pace. Look at young lovers, too—they tend to be masters of synchrony: strolling step in step, holding hands, slow dancing. Synchrony is so powerful, in fact, that coordinating your actions with a complete stranger can make you as empathic toward that person as you would be toward a dear friend.

Laughing with others can also work as social grooming—it elevates pain thresholds and releases oxytocin and endorphins. It's enough to just watch a comedy with a friend for the high-powered bonding to begin. Dunbar argues that dining in company is also a type of synchrony, giving us an endorphin kick and strengthening relationships.

Yet we don't eat with others often enough. One survey has found that a mere 24 percent of Americans in their thirties and forties eat dinner with their family day after day, and it wasn't even specified in the data whether these people dine together at a table or whether everyone shovels in the food while watching TV. In Canada, 70 percent of people admit to watching TV while eating, while almost a third of adult Britons eat alone "most or all of the time." Among middle-aged French people, 61 percent eat dinner with their family, at the table, each and every evening. Americans live on average almost two years shorter than the French. Could there be at least some link in there?

If you really can't make that family dinner happen every night, there is one more, rather subtle way in which matching your movements with another person can make you feel more social, lower your cortisol levels, and directly affect your health. It's called mimicry. Although you might have been told as a child that copycatting others is rude, the truth is we all do it. All the time. We automatically mimic body postures, foot shaking, playing with pens, and facial expressions. And the more empathic someone is, the more they act like a human chameleon.

Have you ever noticed how some married couples start resembling each other after many years down the marital path? Like Tom Brady and Gisele Bündchen? That's a result of mimicry, too. In one experiment people were presented with a pile of pictures—individual portraits of husbands and wives, some from their wedding day and some taken twenty-five years later. The task was to guess who was married to whom. When it came to the photos of the big day, the volunteers just couldn't do it, yet with the silver anniversary images, the success rate was very high. The happier the couple was, the easier it was to match their pictures.

The reason behind this marital doppelgänger effect is that after years of automatically mimicking each others' smiles and frowns, our facial muscles change from all the use and disuse. And the more we play chameleons, the better we feel. Like empathy, mimicry makes us more pro-social, boosts trust, and keeps our blood cortisol low.

What about Botox, then—could it potentially shorten your life? Facial expressions can trigger or change emotions—it's called facial feedback—and studies show that this process malfunctions in people who get Botox injections. Due to the paralysis of some facial muscles, they can't frown or smile properly and find it difficult to mimic or identify the feelings of others. We know from observations of people with Parkinson's disease that those with facial rigidity have trouble keeping friends. Research on chronic anger suppression, meanwhile, suggests that not showing how mad you are by frowning or scrunching your nose can lead to cardiovascular problems. So far there is not enough data on Botox and health to suggest how large the effects might be. Yet the early indications of potential issues are certainly there.

Assuming you haven't had a radical Botox treatment, mimicry can be practised and improved. In preparations for experiments, research assistants are often trained to mimic other people. They are told to wait a couple of seconds and then do a slight variation on the behaviour of the other person. For example, if Mr. A touches his ear, the research assistant may scratch his head. If Mr. A crosses his leg at the ankle, the research assistant might cross it at the knee. It's a skill you can learn—and you may end up more liked and trusted by others, with better relationships. Just be warned: running behind your boss and copycatting every tiny gesture she makes will not get you a promotion (more like get you fired). Becoming a human mirror is not the goal here. Mimicry, like drinking red wine, can be good for health—if practised in moderation.

⧗

To live long, you need strong social relationships. You need a committed romantic partner, a few best friends, and caring neighbours. Whether you will get these relationships depends partially on your luck and life circumstances, but you can also considerably up your chances of a socially included life by developing certain basic qualities: empathy and a secure attachment style. If you test yourself and find out that you are insecurely attached, consider therapy—that's the best way to change your attachment style. But even simply knowing that these things can be changed may push you the first step in the right direction.

As for empathy, you can practise it the way you might practise tennis or yoga: the more you do it, the better you will become. Try to see the world through the eyes of another person at least once a day. Study their facial expressions and body language. Listen, really listen, to what they are saying. Talk to your neighbours, to fellow shoppers in the checkout line, to your waiter—and the more different these people appear from you the better. Watch movies and read books that are particularly good at portraying the world from another person's perspective. Try a human library—a place where people are "books" you can "borrow" and talk to. Some of the "books" are refugees, while others are HIV carriers, deaf-blind people, or soldiers with post-traumatic stress disorder.

You can also groom your social bonds by following the example of our hominin ancestors and using synchrony. Sign up for a choir. Sing with your family more often, no matter how badly. If you want to double the health benefits of exercise, choose sports that can be practised in synchrony, such as group jogging, rowing, or spinning. Make a habit of eating with others—dinners with some alcohol involved (in moderation!) are best, Dunbar tells me. Try to mimic the body language and expressions of people around you, tuning in better into their experiences.

Even if your initial reason for fixing your attachment style, practising empathy, or social grooming is simply your own longevity, the side effects can be quite potent. If we were all securely attached and more empathic, it would not only boost our individual relationships and health, it could also make our planet healthier, too—both socially and environmentally. If we cared more about how our actions impact others, if we were more tolerant and open-minded, there would be less discrimination, less conflict, and less greenhouse gas dumped thoughtlessly into the atmosphere. Think about it: you can prolong your life and make the world a better place in one go.

And when you translate your empathy into sympathy, action directed at improving the lives of others, volunteering, and simple, everyday kindness, your health may profit even more.

A FEW SUGGESTIONS TO BOOST YOUR LONGEVITY

Check your attachment style. If you find it's insecure, consider therapy: secure attachment style is directly linked to better health. Next, work on your empathy—the perfect anti-loneliness drug. Watch empathy-boosting movies and read empathy books. Each day, try to put yourself in other people's shoes. Forget Botox. Turn off your phone. Take empathy classes and sign your kids up for them.

Do things in synchrony with others. Sing and dance. If you do sports, choose ones you can do in sync with friends, such as jogging, rowing, or spinning.

8

HELPING OTHERS
HELPS YOUR HEALTH

Superheroes, UNICEF, and Random Kindness

ERIC HEFFELMIRE WAS IN the garage tinkering underneath his silver GMC Sierra when the jack propping up the car suddenly slid out. The massive frame of the truck pressed Eric to the floor, crushing his chest and shoulders. Small sparks flew off the car and ignited gas that had been leaking from an old freezer. Flames burst up, sending noxious clouds of black smoke into the air.

It was then that the garage doors swung open and Eric's nineteen-year-old daughter, Charlotte, stormed inside. Shocked by the sight ahead she ran toward the truck, grabbed its front, lifted it, and freed her father, saving his life. Somehow the slender five-foot-six teenager managed to hoist the five-thousand-pound truck. "It was some crazy strength," she recalled later, in an interview for a local Virginia radio station.

Stories of such superhuman strength, known as "hysterical strength," are not uncommon. In Oregon, two teenage sisters managed to heft a three-thousand-pound tractor off their father. In Quebec, Lydia Angiyou, a middle-aged mother, fought a polar bear to save her young son and his friends. In Kansas, thirty-something

Nick Harris lifted a Mercury sedan off a neighbour's six-year-old daughter. The list goes on. Although these superhero people usually just prop the bulky vehicles a little off the ground, they still end up lifting hundreds of pounds. Meanwhile, the current deadlift world record—set, by the way, by the actor who played "the Mountain" in *Game of Thrones*—is a "mere" 1,041 pounds. How is it possible, then, that an ordinary teenage girl can suddenly appear as strong as the Mountain? The answer lies most likely in the extra physical power we get from helping others in need, and when that need is particularly great, so is the extra power. After rescuing his young neighbour, Nick Harris tried lifting cars without the added motivation of saving anyone's life and discovered he couldn't.

Most of us don't find ourselves in situations when we need hysterical strength to help others, but even everyday kindness or volunteering for a local charity can boost our physical capabilities and, as a result, our health. The first inkling that caregiving improves fitness came, unexpectedly, from a 1950s study of housewives. Assuming that parenting equals stress and that more stress equals earlier death, researchers from Cornell University followed over four hundred mothers to see whether the most fertile ones would also live the shortest lives. Yet not only did the scientists fail to discover such a connection, they stumbled on another powerful health driver—volunteering. Over the course of the study, half of the women who didn't belong to a volunteer organization fell victim to a major illness. Among those who volunteered, that number was just 36 percent. The researchers were intrigued.

By now we have a hefty pile of studies documenting how powerful benevolence can be for our centenarian potential. Controlling for things such as marital status, religiosity, or social connections, volunteering reduces mortality by 22 to 44 percent—about as much as eating six or more servings of fruits and vegetables each day. What's more, volunteers may have 29 percent lower risk of high blood glucose, about 17 percent lower risk of high inflammation levels, and spend 38 percent fewer nights in hospitals than do people who shy from involvement in charities.

These effects are not restricted to rich countries, either; they show up in places as diverse as Kuwait, Malawi, Kyrgyzstan, and Bolivia. Of course, one could argue that maybe people who are in better health to begin with are simply more likely to pick up volunteering. Imagine signing up for work at a soup kitchen with flared-up arthritis. Yet studies that control for initial health confirm the wellness benefits of volunteering. And if that isn't enough, there are plenty of lab experiments to explain the specific biological mechanisms through which helping others boosts our health.

What Parenting and Cigarettes Have in Common

In 1961, Michio Ikai of the University of Tokyo and Arthur Steinhaus of George Williams College, Illinois, conducted an unusual trial— it involved firing guns near unsuspecting volunteers who signed up for the study. Each of the study's subjects was seated in an armchair, one person at a time, with one of their wrists fastened to the chair with a special belt. They were instructed to pull against the belt as hard as they could whenever the second hand of a clock in front of them crossed the one o'clock position. And so they did, again and again. Then, on one of the attempts, an experimenter would hide behind the armchair and pull out a .22-calibre starter's gun. Right before the volunteer was to strain against the wrist belt, the scientist would fire the gun, startling the unlucky person seated in front of him.

When Ikai and Steinhaus analyzed the data, they discovered that the shock of gunfire pushed up the strength of volunteers by an average of 10 percent. Obviously, 10 percent extra power is still a far cry from being able to tilt a five-thousand-pound truck off a relative. It's just that when you find your loved ones in danger, the hormonal boost your muscles receive is far more massive than in a scenario involving a researcher wielding a starter's gun. The mechanisms, however, are likely the same: they involve the stress response and our evolved caregiving system.

Humans like to pretend we are unique in truly caring for others. As the Dutch primatologist Frans de Waal said in his book *The Age of Empathy: Nature's Lessons for a Kinder Society*:

> People willfully suppress knowledge most have had since childhood, which is that animals do have feelings and do care about others. How and why half the world drops this conviction once they grow beards or breasts will always baffle me, but the result is the common fallacy that we are unique in this regard.

In reality, altruism and helping behaviours are far from rare in the animal kingdom. Just google "animals saving other animals" and your screen will be flooded with cute videos of hippos rescuing drowning baby zebras, horses feeding their hungry neighbours, and baboons chasing off leopards to save antelopes (warning: procrastination danger). If that's not enough to convince you, rest assured that proper scientific studies also find genuine altruism in many animal species, from capuchin monkeys and chimpanzees to ravens and rooks. Rats, for instance, will jailbreak their mates out of their cages even if it means delaying getting to treats as tempting as chocolate chips — and having to share them.

Yet there do exist some evolutionary reasons why human altruism should differ from that of other species. One popular hypothesis states that caring for others developed from parenting behaviours. Since human babies are born particularly vulnerable (thank you, big brains), they require unusually high amounts of care—just ask any under-slept new parent. To ensure that mothers and fathers won't abandon these little needy creatures, nature equipped us with two systems: one reward-inducing and the other stress-reducing.

Jim Jefferies, an Australian comedian, once summed up the experience of parenthood in the following way: "I love my son! I love my son the same way that I love cigarettes. I like to hold him for five minutes every hour, and the rest of the time, I'm thinking about how he's fucking killing me." Jefferies might have been on to something. Neurobiologically speaking, caring for others seems to tap into some of the same brain reward systems as tobacco.

Snug in the middle of our brain is a grape-sized area known as the insula. If you are a smoker and you want to blame something for your addiction to Marlboros or Camels, blame your insula. What's more, damaging that little grape of brain tissue would also quite likely put an end to the habit. Besides addictions, other things that turn on the insula are helping others, donating money to charity, and yes, you've guessed it, caring for kids. Additional reward-related brain areas, the septal area and ventral striatum—the very same ones that light up when you find a winning scratch-and-win card—also buzz with more activity when you take care of others. By wiring parenthood to the reward system, nature assured we wouldn't run screaming from poopy diapers—at least not permanently.

To make caregiving a bit easier still, evolution also linked it with mechanisms that dampen stress. That works in homo sapiens and other animals alike. For female macaques, grooming their mates lowers the levels of stress hormones as measured in the groomers' feces. For elderly human volunteers, caring for infants reduces cortisol levels in the saliva (which could translate into health benefits for the seniors). In general, the more stress people experience in their daily lives, the more beneficial influence helping others exerts on their cortisol.

One way in which caregiving may inhibit stress is through dampening the activity of the amygdala, the fear centre, and disrupting its connections with the fight-and-flight response. Remember the fearless woman called "SM" whom I described in chapter 2? The one who, due to her busted amygdala, was so lacking in fear that she walked up to an obviously sketchy-looking man in a deserted park at night? Although to my knowledge no one has researched SM's levels of benevolence, I wouldn't be surprised if she were particularly into volunteering or donations—people with damaged amygdalae tend to be do-gooders more often than the rest of us.

What's more, when animals hear the whimpers of infants of the same species, the activity of their amygdalae tempers down, too, allowing them to care for the little ones without being freaked out by these weird, needy creatures. Same thing happens with us. Show parents a photo of their baby and their fear centres quiet down like a newborn with a pacifier. The reward-centre septal area may also inhibit the stress response through its action on the HPA axis and the sympathetic nervous system. All in all, helping others calms us down. This dampening of stress in caregiving makes biological sense. To be able to properly care for someone else, you have to take a deep breath and step back from your own issues. Also, to help others in distress, you simply can't be too affected by their suffering. Otherwise your anxiety could make your hands shake and muddle your thinking.

Activating the caregiving system—whether by volunteering at a soup kitchen or by doing shopping for a neighbour—could also boost health through affecting the vagus, that long snake of a nerve bundle that connects your brain, heart, and gut, and which calms down your body after stress, helping you relax. In a way, the vagus is also the nerve of compassion and caring. Have you ever felt your heart go all warm when you saw a puppy rescued from a shelter or heard some uplifting story of human altruism? That was likely your vagus turning on. When people engage in activities that make them experience compassion, the activity of their vagus goes up, too—which could help keep the nerve in shape. And as you may recall from chapter 3, a vagus in tip-top condition keeps your fight-and-flight response in check and your heart rate variability high (a good thing).

Down the road, this altruism-related turning down of the stress response has an impact on our immune systems and inflammation. People who frequently volunteer have lower levels of C-reactive protein—a marker of inflammation. If your blood is teeming with C-reactive protein that's a bad sign, suggesting you may be headed toward developing health problems such as cardiovascular disease. Experiments confirm that it's volunteering per se, and not some other characteristic of people who tend to sign up for unpaid work, that keeps inflammation at bay. At one public high school in western Canada, students were divided into two groups. The first group was to volunteer at a nearby public elementary school helping kids in after-school programs. The second group was wait-listed. When blood samples from all the teens were compared, a clear image emerged: those who had already volunteered had significantly lower levels of an inflammatory marker called interleukin 6. And yes, elevated levels of interleukin 6 are generally bad for you—they can even mean double the risk of dying within the next five years.

Although caregiving in general reduces stress, superhero-style car-lifting works in the opposite way, yet still on the same systems: the amygdala and the fight-and-flight response. Admittedly, it's basically impossible to see what's happening in the bodies of people in the midst of hysterical strength—no ethics commission would approve experiments involving placing people's loved ones under cars. Yet the likely explanation of the superhero effect lies in the workings of the sympathomedullary pathway—the fear-shaken amygdala sending a message down to the adrenal glands, which flood the body with adrenaline, amplifying the power of the hero's muscles.

Besides these outright physiological changes that helping others may elicit—buffering stress, lowering inflammation, or boosting the vagus nerve—volunteering can improve health indirectly. It can make you more socially engaged and help you find new friendships. It can fill your life with meaning and purpose. And, rather prosaically, it can get you off the couch and keep you moving.

But what if getting off the couch is not a problem for you? Maybe instead you wish you could spend more time on the said couch instead of running around the whole day, working, taking care of the kids, the house, the everything? What if you simply can't imagine finding enough time for handing out leaflets on deforestation in the Amazon? The good news is that monetary donations, informal caregiving, and even simple, everyday kindness work well for our health, too.

What Would You Do If You Found $20?

When Lara Aknin was about eight years old she used to trick her younger brother out of his allowance. She would tell him that Canadian nickels were worth more than dimes, because they were bigger, and in every other scenario bigger coins meant more money. She would then have him trade his dimes for her nickels. "He thought he was getting a steal of a deal," she recalls, laughing. "I ended up with double my money and would walk down the street to our corner store and buy all this candy with it. I was really motivated by candy." Years later, when Aknin was doing her PhD in social psychology, she realized that besides being ethically dubious, her childhood thinking was all wrong. Her eight-year-old self would have turned out far happier had she used the dimes to treat her brother instead of herself. By now, Aknin has spent over a decade doing research at Simon Fraser University, British Columbia, proving that although people believe we gain the most happiness from buying stuff for ourselves, in reality we end up better off if we lavish money on others.

Imagine you've found $20 on a deserted sidewalk, so there's no point looking for the owner. What would you do with it? Buy yourself some fancy chocolates? Give the lucky find to a beggar? In one experiment, Aknin and her colleagues handed volunteers either a $5 bill or a $20 bill, then instructed half of the participants to blow the windfall on their own pleasures and the other half to go spend the gift on someone else. Later in the day, once the money had been spent and everyone's moods had been carefully evaluated, Aknin discovered that those who used the money to please others ended up significantly happier than the rest.

It's easy to see how the Bill Gateses of the world might derive psychological benefits from donating their fortunes. Curiously, however, the connection between donations and happiness holds true even for those of us who struggle to have enough dough on a daily basis. When Aknin analyzed pro-social spending across the globe and ran it against happiness levels, she found that the more money inhabitants of a particular country give to others, the more they end up satisfied with life. This was as true in rich nations such as Australia or Germany as it was in poorer ones, such as Ethiopia, Algeria, and Afghanistan.

To confirm the finding, Aknin went back into the lab. She randomly assigned volunteers from two countries, Canada and South Africa, to either purchase a goody bag filled with treats for themselves or to get one for a sick child at a local hospital. Once again, those who spent money on others ended up feeling happier—even though a fifth of South Africans participating in the study reported that sometimes they didn't have enough money to buy food.

Yet a pleasant mood is not the only benefit we may derive from treating others. The gains can be as varied as better sleep, better hearing, stronger muscles, and lower blood pressure. When seniors suffering from hypertension were handed $40 per week for three consecutive weeks to either spend on themselves or on someone else, those who donated the bonus saw their blood pressure drop as much as if they had picked up a healthier lifestyle or started some new medication. And guess what—no side effects!

Charity can also make your muscles stronger. If you are about to try your strength at arm wrestling or would like to impress someone at the gym, just go online first and give $10 or $20 to a charity. In one such experiment, scientists stopped passersby near a subway station in Boston asking if they'd like to try their muscles with a five-pound weight. The task was to hold the weight away from the body, with a fully extended arm, for as long as possible. After the first attempt, the participants were given a dollar, and half were asked if they'd like to donate it to UNICEF. Then everyone was asked to try themselves with the weight once again. The second results were improved—but only for people who had donated the money. Those who gave away their dollar could hold the weight 15 percent longer than those who kept the money to themselves. This may not be as impressive as lifting a GMC Sierra, but still (and no, donating $100,000 won't make you Schwarzenegger-strong in an instant—sorry). The researchers behind the experiment, which was aptly named "The Power of Good," concluded that simply thinking of ourselves as moral people boosts our physical strength.

Besides reaching into your wallet or signing up for formal volunteering, what can also boost your health is caring for those in need in your own family. It may seem counterintuitive that, say, nursing an ailing parent could make us physically better off, as caregiving often involves broken nights, back-breaking labour, and psychological strain. Indeed, a widely cited study from 1999 showed that those who reported strain from caring for their disabled spouses were as much as 63 percent more likely to die within four years than were other people their age.

As years passed, however, more and more research started questioning the assumption that caregiving is always a longevity-wrecker. At least seven large studies have recently shown that many caregivers actually live longer, not shorter. In one such analysis, scientists carefully matched over 3,500 family caregivers with more than 3,500 people who didn't nurse anyone, and discovered that the former had 18 percent lower mortality rates than the latter. That's a comparable effect to that of stuffing yourself with at least 5.8 ounces (165 g) of broccoli and arugula each and every day—and so much more gratifying. As one of the authors of the 1999 study told me, it seems that nursing others may be bad only for a select subgroup of caregivers, such as those who are very old and frail themselves. If you are a grandparent, and not too frail, a great way to foster your health is to babysit your grandkids. Offering such help, assuming it's just an occasional thing and not stepping into the parents' shoes completely, can lower mortality by as much as 37 percent—more than regular exercise (and if your grandkids are small, exercise is inherent in babysitting anyway).

Although large, selfless acts like tending to infirm relatives can lower stress levels and boost health, so can small, everyday acts of kindness—an effect I decided to check for myself. I contacted two scientists at the Stress, Psychiatry and Immunology Lab at King's College, London—Carmine Pariante, a professor of biological psychiatry, and Naghmeh Nikkheslat, a post-doctoral researcher—and they generously agreed to help me out. We discussed the details of my little "experiment," and soon a package with a stamp from King's arrived in my mailbox. Inside, I found simple printouts to be filled out on each day of my intervention and a stash of small plastic tubes called salivettes. For seven days, I was to collect my saliva in the tubes, morning, noon, and evening, and then ship them back to Pariante and Nikkheslat, who would measure my cortisol levels. Four of the saliva-collection days would be just my regular routine days. But the remaining three would be different—on these days on top of everything I normally did, I would add small acts of kindness. These would be my "intervention days."

And so I woke up on day 1 at 7:40 a.m. and groggily reached for the salivette prepared on my night table. I unscrewed the blue cap and slid a roll-shaped swab into my mouth. I was supposed to chew on the swab for a full two minutes to collect enough saliva for testing, and let me tell you, those two minutes seemed never-ending. Rolling the increasingly soggy piece of cotton around my mouth felt disgusting. I gagged. I chewed. I gagged some more. Then I grudgingly repeated the procedure around noon and at 8 p.m. On top of all the chewing, I dutifully noted my moods and everything that happened that day in a journal. Next day, same thing.

The third day was different, though—it was time for my first kindness intervention. As I sat down at my desk planning what fun things I could do for others, I felt my spirits lifting. I scribbled down a long list, specifying things I could do for my husband, for my neighbours, and for strangers. The implementation phase was even more fun. I left a smiley-face sticky note on my neighbours' car. I bought and delivered a small box of chocolates for the nice lady at our local library. At a grocery store, I rushed to open the doors for an elderly woman with a heavy shopping bag. And in the evening I left five-star Google Maps reviews for all my favourite local restaurants and services—something I just hadn't thought of doing before. I don't know whether my telomeres got longer and whether my cortisol response was more healthy, but I certainly felt better, happier. In the evening, as I lay in bed, I was not only calm and content, but also excited for the following day and all the kind things I was planning to do. Broccoli has never given me this feeling, that's for sure.

Over the next two days I continued with random kindness. I bought sandwiches for a homeless family. I donated books. I baked cookies for my husband to take to work and share with his colleagues. I fed stray cats. I picked up trash around my neighbourhood. And I felt good—really good. I had all this extra energy and a bounce in my step. What's more, I was simply having fun.

When the seven days of my "experiment" were up, I stuffed the salivettes into an envelope and mailed them back to London. Two weeks later or so I received news from Nikkheslat: they had the results, and they were exciting. She sent me several pages of numbers and graphs and we set up a call so that she and Pariante could explain to me what this all meant.

Here is what they told me: while on my regular days I produced on average 64 nmol/L of cortisol, on my kindness days I produced just a little under 54 nmol/L, suggesting lower levels of stress. Then Pariante and Nikkheslat went on to explain the numbers day by day (you can find the detailed graphs on this book's website). They pointed out, for instance, how on my first day of random kindness I woke up with quite elevated cortisol levels, which then dropped significantly by noon—by which time I'd already started my acts of kindness. Although cortisol levels normally drop in healthy adults between morning and evening, my drop on that day was quite significant. What's more, the following two "intervention" days, I woke up with considerably lower cortisol levels than I did on regular mornings, as if I were more calm. I found that quite remarkable, especially considering that on day 3 of kindness, I felt particularly jittery and anxious because of political developments in France (the "*gilets jaunes*" protests were in full swing). Yet my body produced less cortisol than on a typical, boring day—it seemed as if my acts of kindness offset the stress of following the news.

Although my seven-day "experiment" was by no means scientific (it had a sample size of one, to begin with), its results did fit into a larger pattern emerging from real, randomized experiments: acts of kindness can improve health by reducing stress and inflammation. In one such "real" experiment in which university students carried out acts of random kindness over the course of three weeks, almost 60 percent claimed to be less stressed as a result. In another, daily volunteering was shown to buffer daily stresses and lower cortisol output (a bit like kindness acts did for me during the "*gilets jaunes*" protests).

Even more convincingly, you can see the effects of kindness in the blood. In one South California study, participants who were assigned to conduct random acts of kindness had their leukocyte genes less tuned toward inflammation. That's a good thing, since chronic inflammation has been linked to such conditions as rheumatoid arthritis, cancer, heart disease, and diabetes. Kindness may also boost health in more extreme circumstances. After a stem cell transplant, many patients suffer from physical issues such as head-aches or nausea. Yet when such patients are asked to write kind let-ters to people who are awaiting a transplant, providing them with advice and encouragement, their symptoms considerably lessen.

What's more, random kindness seems far more contagious than other health behaviours. Take what happened in December 2012 in Winnipeg, Manitoba. At a drive-through of Tim Hortons, someone paid for the meal of the driver behind. Then, that second driver, out of gratefulness, paid for the next person. On and on it went until as many as 228 consecutive cars paid it forward. I have yet to see healthy eating spread with the same fervour.

Pop-up Gardens and the Limits to Volunteering

If you commit your acts of kindness in your own neighbourhood, the benefits may be twofold—even if we are talking longevity only. For one, you may get the regular health benefits of everyday altru-ism, and second, with kindness spreading around, you may end up living in a tight-knit community. That, too, is as vital for physi-cal well-being as is a wholesome diet. Remember Roseto, the little Pennsylvania town where people used to be so resistant to cardio-vascular disease that researchers coined the term "Roseto effect" to describe the phenomenon?

Neighbours in Roseto were particularly welcoming and friendly toward their fellow Rosetans. As one housewife recalled, "We talked. We knew what was going on there and there was always someone around to help you and to keep you from feeling lonely." Studies confirm that to stay healthy we should all live in Rosetos of the world. Take diabetes, for instance. In communities with high social cohe-sion—which is science-speak for trust, willingness to help, and simply getting along with your neighbours—the incidence of type 2 diabetes is 22 percent lower than it is in less friendly places. On the flip side, low social cohesion can mean an increased risk of dying from a heart attack. Even simply having a bad reputation might be enough to make a neighbourhood unhealthy, even if it is unwarranted. The effects of such spatial stigma can be seen in New York City, where inhabitants of areas deemed unwholesome have higher blood pressure than would be justified by their lifestyles or the real characteristics of the 'hood, an effect which has been explained by stress and a lower sense of self caused by living in a stigmatized place.

Unfortunately, most of us reside in places that are no Roseto. In urban Ontario, Canada, only 17 percent of people report a very strong sense of belonging to their community, and in the cities of Alberta and Quebec, that number is as low as 13 percent. In the UK, 84 percent of people don't participate in local events. Americans are not better off—only a quarter even know the names of their next-door neighbours. In my native Poland, meanwhile, gated estates are the problem. After the fall of communism, fences for safety and privacy sprung up everywhere like mushrooms after rain, surrounding both luxurious condominiums and dilapidated apartment buildings. Studies from places as diverse as the US, Malaysia, and Poland itself show that residents of such gated areas report lower sense of belonging. As far as I know, no one has yet compared the longevity of people living in fenced-off neighbourhoods to those in more open spaces, but it would certainly be interesting to see. Does moving to Miasteczko Wilanów, Warsaw, or Beverly Park, Los Angeles, shave years off your life expectancy?

Healthier, closer communities are not just the ones without fences, but also the ones without cars—or at least with fewer of them. The reason for this goes beyond engine noise and tailpipe exhaust. Back in 1969, Donald Appleyard, a British-American urban designer who was fascinated by streets, in particular in their role in the quality of life of local residents, published one of his most famous studies—on traffic and neighbourhood quality. He observed three parallel roads in San Francisco: one that was frequented daily by about sixteen thousand vehicles, which he called Heavy Street; one with eight thousand cars, scooters, or trucks per day, Medium Street; and Light Street, with just two thousand vehicles passing each day. He calculated that residents of Light Street had three times as many friends as those who lived on Heavy Street. They could be often seen sitting on their front steps, chatting with neighbours, while their kids played on the sidewalks. Appleyard didn't check if they lived longer, but chances are, they did.

Should you up and move your family to a quieter community? Maybe, but beware of communities that are too quiet—that is, suburbs. Research shows that children tend to have more friends if they live in geographically flat, walkable areas with plenty of parks and communal spaces. Unfortunately, most American suburbs only meet the "flat" condition, lacking green areas or public squares where children and adults alike can hang out with their friends.

Since for most of us, moving to a peaceful car-free village in rural Italy is out of question, we have to find other ways to make our current neighbourhoods more cohesive, and as such, more longevity-strong. A growing movement called "placemaking" encourages people to reinvent public spaces in their vicinity, which, if done well, should promote a sense of community. Previously shabby vacant lots can be transformed into open gyms and art venues. Main Streets can be closed off to car traffic and pedestrianized. Street markets can be encouraged. Back alleys can be turned into community vegetable gardens. When I lived in Philadelphia, I loved the local tradition of pop-up gardens that in summertime would suddenly appear on street corners or in abandoned parking lots. One day it would be just a weedy, garbage-strewn emptiness, and the next it would metamorphose into a vibrant meeting place, with lush, potted greenery, craft beers on tap, picnic tables, and hammocks.

Placemaking should create a place where residents shop in local stores and chat with neighbours they meet on the way. A place where neighbours not only know each other's names but also visit often.

Where people borrow lawn mowers from each other and water the plants of those who go on holidays. To exist, such a place needs local stores to begin with—so vote for them with your wallet. Say hello to the neighbours you meet as you walk with your groceries (yes, walk, not drive—if that's feasible). Visit your local library and your local playground, even if these are not the best ones in your city. Pick up litter on your street to prevent spatial stigma. The internet is full of ideas on how to placemake your surroundings, some of them quite specific. One of my favourites is having a grill, or even better—a campfire—in your front yard. When Sarah Kobos, a writer for a non-profit called Strong Towns from Tulsa, Oklahoma, bought a cheap fire pit and set it on her front lawn, she discovered that it "attracted people like moths to a flame." She recalls, "Neighbours walked over to see what was going on. People driving by stopped to hang out and chat. Before long, we had to open more wine and bring out the dining room chairs." That's placemaking gone well.

Just as neighbourhoods are not created equal when it comes to their health-promoting effects, the same holds true about volunteering and donations. As Lara Aknin tells me, some ways in which we help others boost our well-being more—and some less. "I think it would be naive to think that every act of generosity is going to pay you the dividend," she says. First and foremost, you need to believe in the cause. Yes, you've heard it right: it's not enough to engage in helping with solely your own health in mind. It may not work. Research shows that people who volunteer for self-oriented reasons, like college applications, don't get the longevity boost from their good deeds. To get effects, we need to activate our biological caregiving system, the one that evolved so that we would help our kin survive. Yet even if you want to pick up volunteering mostly to improve your centenarian potential, don't despair. Aknin believes that it's hard for people to be so completely selfish that they wouldn't be capable of turning on their caregiving systems. Just look deep inside yourself, find things and causes you truly believe in and that can motivate you on a higher level. It may be fighting climate change, improving lives of women in Africa, or supporting a local opera—it doesn't really matter (although Aknin would put a cut-off point before the KKK—if your deepest motivation is hatred for other humans, the longevity benefits would likely not kick in). You can also try developing your empathy and practising compassion meditation, more on which in chapter 10.

When choosing your cause, it's better to pick something where you can easily see the results of your actions. A few years back, Lara Aknin's research assistants walked around the campus of the University of British Columbia asking people if they'd like to donate either to UNICEF or to Spread the Net—an organization affiliated with UNICEF that buys mosquito nets to stop the transmission of malaria. The catch was in the wording of the donation request. While in the case of Spread the Net it said, "Every $10 collected purchases a bed net for a child in Africa—a simple, effective, inexpensive way to make a BIG difference—saving lives, one net at a time," UNICEF claimed, in general terms, to work on "international priorities such as child protection, survival and development." After the donation, the participants were queried on several measures of their well-being. And only people who gave to Spread the Net reaped increasingly more emotional benefits the more they donated—they felt the happiest and the most satisfied with their lives in general.

The explanation for the wellness effects of such targeted support may go back to the workings of the amygdala. If we give money to a needy person we know, rather than to some vague charity cause, our amygdala becomes less reactive to scary things, and our fight-or-flight response calms down. Providing support to others we can identify or easily imagine simply makes us feel more socially connected, which in turns sends a message to our hominin brains that there is no reason to be anxious. In case of trouble, the tribe will protect us.

What that all means in practice is that for your longevity benefits it would be better, for instance, to buy groceries for your poor neighbour than to donate the same amount to a charity that helps some unidentified people. Or that it's better to offer your seat on a bus to a senior in front of you than to sign an online petition for the transportation rights of the elderly. Also, try to frame your helping goals in concrete terms. So no to some abstract "I'll change the world" and yes to "I'll help two kids a month in an after-school program." Even thinking that today you will make someone "smile" is better than assuming you will make someone "happy." This way you will be more able to track your progress and see the results, and results are what boosts well-being.

Another important issue here is freedom—freedom to choose your cause and the extent of your commitment. When my husband worked for a consulting firm in Calgary, Canada, once per year their office participated in a charity event, such as building a house with Habitat for Humanity. It was noble and fun, yet likely didn't benefit my husband's health as much as it would have if he had chosen the cause himself. Simply put, the reward areas of the brain, the ventral striatum and septal area, activate more when we can freely decide to whom and how much to give.

This is why taxes as a form of pro-social spending are likely not as good for health as are voluntary donations, even if the amounts and the recipients are exactly the same. Moreover, perceived lack of choice could also explain why in some cases caring for ailing relatives may be detrimental to the health of the grudging caretaker. And if you want to encourage your kids to help others, avoid rewarding them for their good deeds—not with money, not with stickers. Kids who are promised something in return for volunteering may do the tasks more eagerly at first, but once the carrot is out of sight, their enthusiasm dies down much more than that of children who were never rewarded.

So how much should you donate or volunteer? In terms of financial contributions, it appears that the more the better. Gifts of time are trickier. There is no magic number of hours you should commit to reap the most health benefits—at least none that we know of. It seems that it's best not to overdo on your engagements, as some studies find top wellness returns for under a hundred hours of volunteering per year, while others claim that number is a mere forty.

⏳

We evolved to care. Our do-gooder ancestors, those who nurtured their infants well and who were eager to help others in the tribe—others who knew them and were likely to reciprocate in the future—had higher chances of passing on their genes.

Nature equipped us with systems that encourage giving. Benevolence is hard-wired into the reward areas of our brains, kickstarting the same networks that turn on when we reach for cigarettes or lottery tickets. Helping others also reduces stress, making it easier to offer care and setting off a cascade of physiological changes in our bodies that end up improving our health: reducing blood pressure, lowering inflammation, and, as a result, extending lives.

Although most of us never experience the powerful physical boosts through which altruism can turn us into car-lifting superheroes, we may still profit from the wellness benefits of helping others. Volunteering, random kindness, monetary donations, and caregiving—all these promote longevity at least as well as do exercise and nutritious diets, especially if you do all of them together (studies confirm the effects are cumulative). Find a charity you care deeply about and offer to help them with your time. Donate money to causes you think truly matter. Each day look for opportunities to be kind to others. Although treating yourself to an organic matcha latte could have some positive effects on your physical well-being, you'd likely benefit more by buying it for a friend at work and leaving it on her desk, no strings attached. As my own experiment has taught me, kindness can not only make us feel happier, it can also lower the levels of cortisol circulating in our bodies to calm down everyday stresses.

Of course, the health-boosting effects of random kindness or volunteering don't mean you can now skip your hypertension medications or feast on junk food as much as you want and then just pick up litter in your neighbourhood to counter the damage. In a perfect scenario, you should still eat your five fruits and vegetables a day, do thirty minutes of physical activity Monday through Sunday, and volunteer, donate, and engage in kindness. But life is rarely perfect, so sometimes it may be easier to skip the gym and instead just do a few nice things for the people around you.

You can also try longevity multitasking and choose activities that combine exercise and volunteering (walk dogs for a local shelter, perhaps?) or kindness (stand up in a bus to give your place to someone else). Helping others is such a powerful health improvement tool—maybe one day we will see an official daily recommendations of benevolence? Maybe: "Perform three kind acts a day" or "Volunteer or care for others for a minimum of thirty minutes per week"? Certainly seniors could already profit from public health policies that would encourage them to engage in charitable work, preventing social isolation and physical decline—and, from a budgetary perspective, quite on the cheap, too.

Admittedly, the idea of picking up random kindness or volunteering simply for their health benefits might make some people cringe. But, as mentioned above, if some theoretical do-gooders were solely motivated by a selfish concern for longevity, their biological caregiving systems would likely not activate anyway and the health benefits wouldn't materialize. It's okay, though, both biologically and, as I believe, ethically, if the first impulse to rethink your helping behaviours comes from an egoistic desire to live longer. If it makes you take a closer look at how you contribute to your community and how you spend your money and time, and makes you commit more to altruism, both society and your body should profit in the long run. It may not be very idealistic, but it sure works. Here is a more idealistic thought, though: contrary to other health behaviours, philanthropy is very contagious, so by giving to others you will not only live longer, but you may also end up spending the extra years in a slightly better, kinder world.

For some of us, stepping up the do-good effort may be relatively easy. You may already be volunteering or donating money regularly. But in case your caregiving system does get a bit rusty, luckily there are ways to rev it up. One such trick involves working on changing your personality, since conscientious and extroverted people tend to volunteer more. And yes, personality can indeed be tweaked—with health benefits.

A FEW SUGGESTIONS TO BOOST YOUR LONGEVITY

Activate your evolved caregiving system: donate to charity, care for others in your family, and volunteer for causes you truly believe in, be it investing in art, fighting rare diseases, or protecting the environment. Engage in every-day kindness—open doors for others, buy a coffee for a stranger, or leave a friendly note on a random car's windshield. Placemake your community: encourage opening of community gardens and vote for pedestrianization of main streets. Shop in local stores, walk around, pick up litter, and talk to your neighbours.

9

WHY PERSONALITY
AND EMOTIONS MATTER
FOR LONGEVITY

Don't Worry, Be Happy—
and Organize Your Sock Drawer

ON SEPTEMBER 22, 1930, Mother Mary Stanislaus Kostka, a plump, round-faced nun who was at the time the North American superior of the School Sisters of Notre Dame, sent a letter to the convents requesting that each novice write a short autobiography before taking her final vows. Soon, the handwritten life accounts started to pile up. And even though they were supposed to be concise and contain quite specific information (place of birth, school attendance, parentage), the biographies differed considerably in their delivery. One sister wrote, "God started my life off well by bestowing upon me a grace of inestimable value . . . The past year which I have spent as a candidate studying at Notre Dame College has been a very happy one. Now I look forward with eager joy to receiving the Holy Habit of Our Lady and to a life of union with Love Divine."

Another young nun, meanwhile, recounted, "I was born on September 26, 1909, the eldest of seven children, five girls and two boys . . . My candidate year was spent in the Motherhouse, teaching Chemistry and Second Year Latin at Notre Dame Institute. With

God's grace, I intend to do my best for our Order, for the spread of religion and for my personal sanctification."

The differences between the two passages may be subtle, yet when you look at them more carefully, you may notice that the first nun's writing is loaded with positive emotion. She writes about "a very happy" year and about her "eager joy." The second woman, on the other hand, is more subdued in her accounts, dryly stating facts. For health and longevity, such differences matter. Many decades after Mother Kostka sent her call for autobiographies, three University of Kentucky researchers went into the convent's archives and dug out handwritten bios of 180 nuns. They carefully analyzed the accounts, coding each word as either emotionally positive, negative, or neutral. Gratitude, hope, and relief would be marked as positive, for instance, while anger, disgust, and fear as negative. The scientists also checked which of the nuns were still alive, and at what age the others had passed away. The results were pretty clear: these sisters who were the most joyful and optimistic in their autobiographies were also the ones who lived the longest. Sunny disposition meant on average an additional ten years of life.

It's not just nuns who reap longevity benefits from having a positive outlook—so do famed psychologists and orangutans. A decade after the convent study, a similar analysis of autobiographies of deceased psychologists, including such stars as B. F. Skinner and Jean Piaget, showed a connection between a penchant for using positive words and reaching an impressively advanced age. In zoos, meanwhile, happy orangutans are long-lived orangutans. And no, memoir-writing apes have not yet been discovered. Instead, zoo keepers in forty-two parks across the globe were asked to evaluate their charges, for example indicating how often each animal seems to experience positive versus negative moods. Once again the longevity differences were striking: about eleven extra years for the happy apes.

Humanity has long suspected that happiness extends lives. Already the Bible states that "the joyfulness of man prolongeth his days"

(Ecclesiasticus 30:22), and according to Shakespeare, "Mirth and merriment . . . bars a thousand harms and lengthens life." Science is now catching up with literature. Among over ten thousand academic publications that come out each year on the topic of subjective well-being, many are finding that positivity equals better health and a better shot at becoming a centenarian. It appears that happiness can add anywhere from four to ten years of life. One particularly well-done British study, in which existential enjoyment was measured every two years for six years in total, concluded that people who each time reported feeling full of energy, enjoying everyday things, and looking back on their life with a sense of happiness were 24 percent less likely to die than were their less cheerful peers.

But maybe it's just that being in poor physical shape simply makes people miserable, and if you are in poor physical shape you die early—logical, right? However, such cause-and-effect issues can be fairly easily controlled for by taking into account initial levels of health when happiness is measured, and checking the physiological outcomes years down the road. Besides, we also have animal studies and experiments (yes, on humans too) that show that our moods impact our biology—for example by influencing inflammatory processes or DNA methylation.

Here is a thing, however: measuring happiness is a tough job. Are you happier than your parents? Than your neighbours? How do you know? It's not like we can take someone's blood sample and count the joy molecules floating in the serum. Even things like language can affect people's reports of well-being. The French word for feeling happy, "*heureux*," as well as the German "*glücklich*" or Polish "*szczęśliwy*" carry much more weight than does "happy." You wouldn't necessarily say eating ice cream makes you *heureux* or *szczęśliwy* (or it would have to be some freakishly good ice cream). What's more, you may get positive moods from not very kosher sources—like cocaine or magic mushrooms. For these reasons, scientists these days like to talk about something they call "subjective well-being," which basically covers joy, optimism, and general life satisfaction altogether.

To make things even more complicated, many psychologists also differentiate between hedonic and eudaemonic well-being—or in other words, between pleasure and meaning. Here is a thought experiment: imagine you could get connected to a futuristic machine that could make you experience any pleasure known to humans, from the delights of travel to the bliss of love. You would simply spend your days floating in a tank with electrodes connected to your brain, loading on fun. Would you plug in? Would such a life be truly happy?

The scenario in this thought experiment, designed by American philosopher Robert Nozick and hence called Nozick's Experience Machine, has been proposed to hundreds of people in several studies, and in most cases, met with rejection. Somehow we instinctively feel that despite all the pleasures, life in Nozick's machine wouldn't be truly good. One major component that such existence would be missing is eudaemonic well-being: purpose, self-actualization, and a sense of meaning—and although in theory the machine could also simulate such feelings, our instincts go against having meaning in life that's only virtual. Such lack of real purpose, in turn, could make life in Nozick's contraption not only empty, but also short.

It appears that for health and longevity, having meaning in life may be more important than happy moods. In one study that directly compared hedonic and eudaemonic well-being, people with purpose in life had a favourable gene expression pattern related to the fight-or-flight response, while those fixated on the pursuit of bodily pleasures had an unfavourable one. In other words, people who have found meaning in their existence had more good genes turned on and more bad ones switched off. What's more, finding meaning not only boosts our chances of becoming centenarians, it also lowers the risk of cognitive impairment—even in the face of Alzheimer's disease. If a ninety-year-old with a clear purpose in life develops

Alzheimer's disease, they are likely to keep functioning relatively well despite very real pathological changes in the brain.

Finding meaning may be particularly important when "the excrement hits the air conditioning" (to paraphrase Kurt Vonnegut's words from *Hocus Pocus*) or, less poetically, when things don't go as planned. In lab experiments, when purposeful people are made to look at disgusting or disturbing pictures of violence and sickness, their amygdalae stay relatively calm and they recover from the unpleasant experience much faster than do people who don't have much purpose. Friedrich Nietzsche was right when he wrote that "He who has a Why to live for can bear almost any How." Besides, eudaemonic well-being means more grey matter in the insula—the reward-related brain area—and more grey matter in the insula can help us regulate emotions and deal with stress.

One way in which having purpose in life can translate into longevity is through its impact on our health-related behaviours. People who feel their existence has meaning are more likely to get their cholesterol levels checked or to have long rubber tubes inserted into their backsides on a regular basis (colonoscopy). But eudaemonic well-being seems to also have direct impacts on our biology, lowering the levels of cortisol and pro-inflammatory cytokines.

Now for the million-dollar question: how do you become happier and how do you find purpose in life? Many books and scientific papers have been written on the topic, and although no one has found a silver-bullet solution as yet, we do have some indications of what works and what doesn't. I won't go into details—my publisher wouldn't be happy if I submitted a thousand-page book—but here are a few basic research-based tips. First, instead of looking for hedonic pleasures, try to find purpose in your day-to-day life. A good first step is to simply acknowledge that meaning is important and to spend time reflecting on it. Try to recognize your own character strengths and think about how your talents might profit others (in a charitable way). For more ideas, you may want to reach for such books as the classic *Man's Search for Meaning* by Viktor Frankl or the recent *The Power of Meaning: Finding Fulfillment in a World Obsessed with Happiness* by Emily Esfahani Smith.

Second, it's important to remember that extra money is not really a solution, and it won't make you happier. The more people tend to focus on their financial goals, the less happy they become—and this is true not only in the rich countries of the world, but also in the less prosperous ones such as Russia and India. Of course, for people who are struggling to meet their basic needs, a thicker wallet would mean higher well-being, but above a certain income level more dough does not necessarily equal more joy.

Richard Easterlin, a renowned American economist, explained that favourable effects of rising paycheques on well-being get erased because the more we have, the more we tend to want. As Ralph Waldo Emerson once wrote, "Want is a growing giant whom the coat of Have was never large enough to cover." Lab experiments also suggest that when people fixate on money, they become less social and less helpful—and as we know from the links between sociability and health, this could potentially mean lower chances of one day getting that cake with a hundred candles on it. However, there are ways of bagging more happiness out of money. What works, for instance, is buying experiences instead of material goods (so yes to the family trip to an amusement park, no to the newest smartphone). Another thing is spending your bucks on others instead of yourself—donating to charity, lavishing gifts on your loved ones, and so on.

Third, don't chase happiness at all costs—it will keep escaping. Just as with money, fixating on happiness as a goal can backfire and make you less satisfied with life. Remember FOMO from chapter 6? Although the word was only officially added to the *Oxford English Dictionary* in 2013, it's already such a big deal that the Anxiety and Depression Association of America has dedicated a website to overcoming FOMO.

FOMO, or "fear of missing out," is a constant nagging feeling that others are enjoying themselves more, dining in better restaurants, visiting more fun holiday destinations, and going to more hip parties. And that you should be doing these things, too. The Anxiety and Depression Association of America recommends that you try switching off the chatter—so no Facebook or Instagram—and practise savouring simple daily experiences. Instead of fretting that you can't jet off to the Maldives, enjoy camping in a nature reserve near your home. Instead of agonizing over which award-winning chef makes the best oysters in town and why you aren't eating them right now, make the dish at home. But beware: eating raw shellfish could have unexpected consequences for your health and longevity—it could change your personality.

Undercooked Meat, At-Risk Personality and How Worry Can Kill You

It was nighttime. A single lab rat entered his experimental outdoor pen and sniffed at a layer of white sand covering the ground. Ahead of him stretched a brick maze, which he soon started exploring. As he walked around, the rat suddenly came upon a strange smell wafting from one of the labyrinth's corners. He approached with growing curiosity. The scent seemed to pull him in.

What the rat found so alluring that night, as did many of his labmates tested in the maze, was cat urine—something that rats normally consider scary and try to avoid. But this rat was different. Just like several other rodents in this particular experiment, he had been infected with a parasite called *Toxoplasma gondii*. The parasite, as the scientists conducting the trials found out, considerably changed the way the rats behaved. Not only did they display this weird and potentially fatal feline attraction, but they were also more eager to explore the maze than were uninfected rodents.

Humans are no rodents, but *T. gondii* infection may impact our personality as well. According to some studies, once this tiny parasite makes its home in a person's body, that person could become more impulsive, sensation-seeking, and aggressive (there are even some initial suggestions that *T. gondii* increases the risk of having traffic accidents). For a long time, it was believed that personality couldn't change, that once an extrovert always an extrovert, etc. Yet decades of studies have revealed that personality can indeed be altered, and not just by ingesting parasites but by our own efforts, too. That's good news, since personality can have a large impact on health and longevity.

There are five main dimensions of personality, known also as the "big five." You can be either extroverted or introverted, neurotic or emotionally stable, open to experience or closed to it, agreeable or antagonistic, and conscientious or irresponsible. Of course, it's not all or nothing. You can be very extroverted or just a little bit. One person can be far more conscientious than another. That's why researchers usually talk about being one or two standard deviations above or below the mean on a certain personality trait. To get a better idea what this might mean, imagine differences in personality as differences in height between people. The contrast between being one or two standard deviations above the mean on, say, introversion, would be like being five feet six inches (168 cm) tall versus six feet tall (183 cm) for an American man.

It's not just humans that differ in personality—animals do too. Spotted hyenas, rats, chimpanzees, and even trout have distinct personality types. And just like in humans, certain personality profiles seem better for animal longevity. Bolder, more aggressive trout have shorter telomeres in their fins than do fish that tend to behave differently. In people, the connection between personality and health is already so well established that some researchers are calling for interventions for personality types they call "at-risk"—something akin to "do at least 150 minutes a week of moderate-intensity exercise." In the case of personality, though, it would more likely be "tidy and plan for 150 minutes a week." That's because the personality type that appears particularly important for health and longevity is conscientiousness—having a penchant for tidying, planning, and preparing.

Have you ever watched the television classic *Gilmore Girls?* The show's main character, Lorelai Gilmore, is charming and sweet but also messy and impulsive. Her diet consists of whatever she suddenly starts craving ("cheeseburger, with a side of cheeseburger, and . . . a cheeseburger smoothie") and about ten litres of coffee per day. If Lorelai were a real person, she would be in longevity trouble. A person two standard deviations below the mean in conscientiousness has a 44 percent higher mortality risk compared to someone two standard deviations above the mean. If you could ingest conscientiousness in a pill, it would be a miracle drug—its effects would be much stronger than those of aspirin on reducing heart disease or the Salk vaccine on polio. The positive effects of being organized and industrious are found all across the planet, including Canada, Japan, and Sweden. And if you have a child whose room resembles a constant post-hurricane zone (I have one of those myself), you should be at least as concerned about the effects this mayhem has on your kid's future health as you may be about their candy intake. Conscientiousness measured in childhood can predict longevity even as far as seven decades into the future.

Part of an explanation for why conscientious people live longer is the fact that they tend to abstain from cheeseburger smoothies, exercise regularly, and follow doctors' advice. As generally more level-headed people, they choose stable friendships, stay married, succeed at work, and wear seat belts. But even if you control for all of the above and many more health-related behaviours, the strong effects of conscientiousness on longevity still persist. Psychologists studying the topic believe direct biological mechanisms are at play, such as the functioning of the immune and nervous systems, but these mechanisms are still not well understood.

Being low on conscientiousness is particularly dangerous when combined with another personality trait, neuroticism. Take most movie characters played by Woody Allen, and you will get what neuroticism is all about (hypochondria meets constant worrying meets frequent low moods). Although the term is often used lightly, being neurotic is not much fun. People high on this personality trait tend to be anxious and tense, perceiving the world around them as threatening and unsafe. They are often unhappy about the way their lives are unfolding and experience quite a lot of negative emotions, including anger, guilt, and sadness. And yes, they tend to be hypochondriacs, too. If the above seems to describe you, you may be in trouble, since being neurotic can mean even 33 percent higher risk of mortality. Again, these effects are only in small part explained by the propensity of neurotic people to smoke, drink alcohol, or have trouble socializing.

Neuroticism is in fact such a health-wrecker that it may have serious impacts on the economy. In the Netherlands, for instance, the top most neurotic people cost the country over $1.3 billion per year per million inhabitants in health services, out-of-pocket costs, and production losses. And the Netherlands is not even among the most neurotic countries—that would be Greece, followed by Russia (although this particular study compared only thirty-seven nations). The least neurotic country proved to be Israel, with the US, UK, and Canada hovering in the middle. In the US, Pennsylvania, Ohio, and New York have the most neurotic people, while Alaska and Arizona have the least.

One of the reasons why neuroticism may be bad for health could be its connection to worry and rumination. Rumination is dwelling on events and emotions, going over and over the same stuff in your head like a cow chewing its cud. Worry is rumination's cousin, but while we usually ruminate about things that have already happened, worry precedes potential stressful events—which, by the way, most often don't materialize. The problem with worriers and ruminators is that their autonomous nervous systems are chronically activated. The stress they experience doesn't affect them only when the bad stuff actually happens, but also well before it does and long after.

This can lead to unfortunate health consequences. People who worry a lot tend to have fewer natural killer cells—lymphocytes that launch attacks against infections and tumours. What's more, worry-prone men who have suffered a myocardial infarction are more likely to get unlucky a second time. And if you are awaiting surgery, worrying about it can make recovery tougher. In one study, patients with hernias who fretted about the procedure the most ended with lower levels of immune cells at the wound site and greater pain. They also took longer to get better.

Just as low conscientiousness and high neuroticism increase the risk of dying prematurely, extraversion seems to lower it—although the links between this personality type and longevity are less well established. Extraversion is associated with about a 21 to 24 percent lower risk of mortality—more or less as much as the Mediterranean diet—but about half of the effect is explained by the extroverts' propensity to socialize (good for health) and exercise (also good for health).

There used to be one more personality type famously linked with health, and with cardiovascular health in particular—the so-called type A personality. You know the sort: constantly looking at their watch, always stressed, irritable, obsessed with work. And yet I'm saying "used to be" and "so-called" because research on the type A personality is passé. Since the initial hype in the 1950s and 1960s, follow-up studies haven't confirmed the effects of the type A personality on heart attacks or clogged arteries. There may have been a good reason for this. In recent years, it came to light that the tobacco industry had been happily funding epidemiological studies on type A behaviours—for example by paying key researchers in the field. Such investments made perfect sense for them. Show that it's not the clouds of inhaled smoke that cause heart disease but instead impatience and workaholism, and you are all set. For the tobacco industry, the type A personality made for a great cardiovascular scapegoat.

However, one ingredient of the type A personality has made a comeback (and no, the tobacco industry is not paying for the research): hostility. If you ever find yourself being cynical, mistrusting others, believing everyone around you is selfish, and responding to stress with aggression—well, don't. Apart from being hard on other people and alienating them, it's bad for your heart. It can cause problems with your triglycerides, your glucose levels, and your insulin resistance. Such behaviours, bunched by psychologists into something they call "hostility," are associated with an increased risk of cardiovascular events—basically, your heart giving up on you. And when it comes to anger not befitting ladies, it looks like grandma may have been right after all, albeit for different reasons than she might have thought. Studies show that hostility is particularly detrimental to women, messing with the inflammatory processes in their bodies, which in turn may lead to cardiovascular disease.

While the type A personality is no longer on the research agenda, there is a new kid on the block: the type D personality. The "D" stands for "distressed," as in: experiencing a lot of negative emotions such as anger, irritability, sadness, and fear, while being unwilling or unable to share these emotions with others to get some relief. Type Ds worry. They get irritated. They feel blue—a lot. As a result, their bodies age faster. They have shorter telomeres, and their inflammatory proteins are as elevated as if they were ten years older than they really are. Type Ds are also prone to having something called "soft" or "vulnerable" plaque, which is a perfect recipe for a heart attack. As opposed to the regular, stable kind of plaque that can clog your arteries, the lipid core of vulnerable plaque is covered only by a thin, fibrous cap—a bit like a garbage bin secured only with foil instead of a sturdy lid. If things go bad, that fibrous cap can break suddenly and erupt like a tiny volcano, with all the accumulated junk suddenly spilling into your artery, causing a heart attack. In a way, this scenario can be more dangerous than the slow buildup of regular plaque, so the fact that type Ds have a 2.5 times increased chance of such volcano-like plaque rupture is a serious matter. They are also almost four times more likely to die than other patients with coronary heart disease. For these very reasons, having a type D personality is now considered a cardiovascular risk factor by the European Cardiovascular Prevention Guidelines.

All that said, what if you are a child of a Lorelai Gilmore type and a Woody Allen type? A neurotic, disorganized pessimist? Other than gorging yourself on undercooked meat or digging through cat feces to get infected with a personality-changing toxoplasmosis parasite, can you somehow alter your nature? The good news is that it can indeed be done, no kitty poop involved. One way to change your personality is to simply . . . wait. Human nature tends to shift with age toward less neurotic, less extroverted, and less open to experience but more agreeable. Conscientiousness is more tricky—first it goes up, then peaks around middle age, and then falls down again in later years. Of course, these are just population averages and won't tell you what will happen to any particular person. For some people, for instance, extraversion can increase with age instead of declining, and so on.

What may speed up the changes in personality are major life events: getting married, becoming a parent, and so on. If you are a married woman, and you've noticed that since the wedding your husband is happy to trade his party outfits for slippers, you are not alone. One study done on over three hundred spouses living in Florida revealed that over the first eighteen months of marriage, new husbands became much less extroverted. For those who find this disturbing, the upside is that said husbands also became more conscientious—that is, more likely to pick up their dirty socks from the bathroom floor. Women, on the other hand, became considerably less neurotic after the vows.

Other life events may also have an impact on personality. There are some reports that divorce increases extraversion in women, getting fired decreases conscientiousness, and joining the military can make you less agreeable. Practice makes perfect, as the saying goes, and since being newly single often forces women to go out more, doing so may increase their extraversion. Jobs tend to require conscientiousness, and losing them make us practise the trait less. Military training, meanwhile, encourages behaviours that don't fit with agreeableness: aggression, for instance. The more we do something, the more we change.

But apart from waiting for love to strike or for Uncle Sam to call, you can take things into your own hands. You can change your personality traits at any age, even a very advanced one, although it is easiest done between the ages of twenty and forty. Some personality dimensions are harder to budge, such as openness to experience. Neuroticism, meanwhile, is the easiest trait to work on, which is good news from the longevity perspective. And here is some more good news: the process doesn't need to take years. Interventions to alter people's personality traits usually work after about eight to twenty-four weeks, depending on the study.

In one particularly thorough study, close to four hundred students from the University of Illinois at Urbana-Champaign and Michigan State University entered a fifteen-week program designed to help them change their personality traits. The whole idea was based on the principle of "fake it till you make it." Each week, the students received a list of challenges to complete on the study website, ranging from very easy ("organize the app icons on your phone's home screen") to more difficult ("ask a co-worker, neighbour, or classmate to lunch or dinner"). They were to pick several tasks off the list—whatever took their fancy. The challenges were customized based on the student's performance the week before: successful completion of several tasks meant the website would suggest slightly more difficult ones the next time. In case of a failure, easier options would pop up on the screen.

It all worked quite well. Students who wanted to increase their extraversion, for instance, and who completed a mere two challenges per week, increased this particular personality dimension by a fifth of a standard deviation over the semester. Using the height comparison, that would be like your average man growing over half an inch (1 cm). Not a tremendous shift, but certainly something. What still remains to be seen, though, is whether such change can be truly long-lasting or perhaps requires regular "reminder" interventions.

If you want to try some personality-shifting challenges at home, this study includes a handy list of tasks you can pick and choose. Just to give you an idea, here are a few examples.

To boost your extraversion:

- Say hello to a cashier at a store.
- Call a friend whom you haven't spoken with in a while.
- Go to a new restaurant or bar and chat with your server.

To work on your conscientiousness:

- Set out your clothes the night before.
- When you notice something you need to buy (e.g., household supplies), make a note on your phone.
- Pay a bill as soon as you receive it.

To diminish neuroticism:

- When you feel overwhelmed, stop and take several deep breaths.
- Before you go to bed, write down one good thing you can look forward to tomorrow.
- When you feel worried about the future, spend at least two minutes visualizing the best-case scenario.

Seems tough? Well, you could always just pop a few magic mushrooms instead. Their active compound, psilocybin, has been shown to shift certain personality dimensions even after a single dose—although admittedly, that particular study was small and has yet to be replicated. One thing is certain, however: just thinking about changing your personality is not enough. You have to actually do something (and I'd strongly suggest going for the behavioural challenges, not the magic mushrooms). The payoffs can be substantial. Changes in personality traits over time are at least as important for longevity as are general levels of extraversion, neuroticism, or conscientiousness. Say there is one man, let's call him Mr. Grumpy, who is quite neurotic, but stays more or less the same throughout his grumpy life. Now, a second man, Mr. Sulky, starts at a relatively lower level of neuroticism in his youth, but increases on the scale quite a lot as the years pass. Who will be worse off? A study of over a thousand American veterans suggested that Mr. Sulky may be in for trouble: increasing levels of neuroticism can push up the risk of dying by 40 percent—more so than the lifestyle of a couch potato.

If you are a parent, and you'd like to set your kids on a centenarian path of not being Mr. or Ms. Grumpy, there are things you can do to help them. For one, don't do what made some parents in Hayward, California, and Darien, Connecticut, end up in the headlines. Elementary schools in Hayward and Darien reported trouble with overzealous moms and dads who swarm school cafeterias at lunchtime to help their offspring deal with the many challenges surrounding the ingestion of soups and burgers—and we are talking kids even as old as ten. The parents bring extra snacks. They solve social troubles. They spoon-feed. These are the masters of helicopter parenting.

Some emerging research is beginning to indicate that helicopter parenting may lead to neuroticism once the kids become young adults. On the other hand, simply being a warm and loving parent without the hovering seems to translate into having children who grow up to be more conscientious and emotionally stable—set on the path to becoming centenarians.

⧗

If you were truly happy with your life you would probably want that life to last as long as possible—and in a lucky biological twist, that's precisely the way nature has arranged it. Those full of joy and those who have found meaning in their existence are the very same people who are the most likely to escape the Grim Reaper. On the flip side, in excess, worrying, rumination, or negative emotions kill us slowly yet steadily.

From the perspective of longevity, personality traits are not created equal—some are simply more conducive to reaching the centenarian years. Extraversion is like that. Conscientiousness is like that. Emotional stability is like that. You could dismiss these effects by saying that a large part of them comes from the way personality influences pro-health behaviours like smoking, diet, and exercise. And it's true—it does.

Yet we shouldn't dismiss personality-changing interventions if we are looking for healthier, longer lives. You could, of course, just focus on each health behaviour individually. Try to eat more whole grains. Try to take more steps each day. Try to cut down on sugar, alcohol, and junk food. But targeting your personality traits is a bit like getting the master key—a key that can be used to regulate all health behaviours in one go. If you become more conscientious, getting diet and exercise right will be less of an uphill battle. Tone down neuroticism, and you will be less likely to calm your nerves with tobacco. Increase your extraversion, and health-boosting social relationships will come more easily to you. And on top of all that, the biological mechanisms that link personality with health may slow down your aging even further.

However, there is a caveat to consider: although personality and emotions do affect average lifespans, we shouldn't blame each and every illness on personality defects. If Mr. A has a heart condition, it doesn't mean he is a miserable neurotic with no purpose in life. There are many reasons for why we get sick, starting with genes and followed by the environment in which we live, and although working on certain personality traits can help boost our immune systems or stave off cognitive decline, it won't make us disease-proof. Nothing can. What personality changes can do for you is simply lower your risks of dying prematurely and suffering ill health.

If you were to pick just one personality trait to work on in order to increase your chances of becoming a centenarian, go for conscientiousness. Fake it until you make it—set yourself small challenges of conscientious things to try and do. Keep your office desk neat. Organize your sock drawer. Set out your clothes the night before.

The next on the list would be tackling neuroticism: worrying less and sharing your problems with others. Therapy is the best way to go if you really want to change. Mindfulness and meditation are also good for neurotic people and their telomeres (more on that in the next chapter). The plus here is that this particular personality trait is quite malleable and the easiest to change.

Last but not least, if you care about your health and longevity don't simply go on chasing hedonistic pleasures. Don't fixate on getting more and more money. Instead, try to find a deeper purpose, a "why" that could help you bear almost any "how." Difficult? If you sit in a quiet spot in a yoga position, breathing mindfully, you may find all these challenges a bit less overwhelming. After all, even rats get more laid-back when they practise yogic breathing.

A FEW SUGGESTIONS TO BOOST YOUR LONGEVITY

If you are neurotic and not very conscientious, try working on these personality traits—it can be done and your health will profit. You can see changes even after a few weeks of simple exercises. Avoid excessive worry and rumination, and if you find yourself being often angry and cynical, talk to a therapist. Although optimism and joy prolong life, don't chase happiness as an ultimate goal. Instead, try to find purpose. Your life will not only be more meaningful for that, but may last longer, too.

HOW MEDITATION AND MINDFULNESS BOOST HEALTH

Slow Breathing, Yoga Rats, and
Horror-Stricken Leukocytes

MAHARISHI MAHESH YOGI, a Hindu monk, looked like an encyclopedia illustration for an entry titled "meditation guru." He had Jesus-like hair, a long, greying beard, and flowing white robes. It's possible, though, that we might imagine meditation gurus in a certain way precisely because that's how Maharishi Mahesh Yogi looked: after all, it was his lecture at the Hilton Hotel in London on August 24, 1967, that gave a great push to the popularity of transcendental meditation in the West. That day, in the front row of an auditorium full of people, sat three special guests: John Lennon, Paul McCartney, and George Harrison (Ringo stayed home with his newborn son).

The Beatles were transfixed by Maharishi's words and decided to pick up meditation right there and then. Six months later, the Fab Four followed Maharishi to his ashram in India to take a deep plunge into transcendental meditation. "The meditation buzz is incredible," Harrison claimed in one interview. "I get higher than I ever did with drugs." In John Lennon's words, meanwhile, "Buddha was groovy."

Although today, few people would call meditation "groovy," mind-body practices certainly haven't lost their popularity. Quite the opposite, in fact. Modern-day celebrities from Katy Perry and Ellen DeGeneres to Hugh Jackman and Oprah Winfrey preach the wonders of mindfulness, while airports all over the planet open dedicated "yoga rooms" for tired travellers. Almost one in five Americans report that they have used at least one mind-body therapy in the past year, and 1.5 million Canadians practise yoga. In England, meanwhile, several hundred schools have recently introduced a new subject to the curriculum: mindfulness.

The benefits of mind-body practices are supposed to be many, from the "classics" such as better sleep and dampening of stress to more unconventional ones like cellulite reduction and increased hair growth. And although to my knowledge no research exists on how meditation could remedy cellulite or make anyone's locks more swishy, a substantial collection of studies does support the notion that mind-body therapies may improve some aspects of health and may even prolong lives. Yes, the studies are still new, and not all findings are conclusive, but some trends are already emerging.

There are many different research-tested mind-body practices, from yoga and meditation to the lesser-known qigong. Among various meditation styles, scientists tend to distinguish three main types: focused attention, open monitoring, and kindness-oriented. Focused attention is the mantra-chanting kind of practice: you stay still and fixate your mind on something, say a word or a candle. If your mind wanders, you bring it back to the point of focus. In open monitoring, on the other hand, you just observe the present moment with everything it brings—your thoughts (need to do laundry), your bodily sensations (that itch in the left toe), accepting everything as it happens.

The last type of meditation, kindness-based, centres on others to develop compassion. It may involve, for instance, directing positive thoughts toward your mail carrier or check-out clerk, or even someone you don't like very much. Within these broad categories lie myriad different meditation styles, from the trendy mindfulness meditation to om meditation, Zen, vipassana, and so on. Some internet sources also suggest dishwashing meditation, labyrinth meditation, and crystal meditation (involving holding various crystals in your hands), but science remains poignantly silent on these ones.

No matter the style, research suggests that mainstream meditation practices make the body's stress axes, the sympathomedullary axis and the HPA, less active—with all its downstream physiological consequences, including those directly implicated in aging.

The fact that the Beatles' yogi, Maharishi, lived to be ninety-one may have had something to do with his ashram-based lifestyle. It appears that even a short stay at a meditation retreat may affect your DNA in a pro-longevity way. In one 2018 experiment, just one month spent at Spirit Rock Meditation Center in Woodacre, California, was enough to stretch out the participants' telomeres by about 104 base pairs, which could be roughly compared to four years of life. Admittedly, the program was intense. Participants were required to engage in various meditation practices for about ten hours per day—all in total silence.

Although it still remains to be seen whether the results of such telomere-extending retreats persist long-term, other studies point in a similar direction. Expert Zen meditators who have practised daily for over ten years have far longer telomeres than do people of the same age who have never meditated. Mind-body therapies may also slow down the ticking of your epigenetic clock: DNA from the blood cells of long-term meditators show changes suggesting that the more you practise, the more slowly you age. And even though staying at hippie California retreats may not necessarily rebalance your chakras, it may change your *FOXO* genes—the same type of genes that are behind the immortality of hydras.

Chanting "om" and practising mindfulness may not only hold back aging, it may also rewire the brain. If you put someone who meditates a lot into a neuroimaging machine, you may see quite pronounced changes in six to eight different brain regions; these could happen through formation of new synapses between neurons in some of the regions and loss of neurons in others. A mere few weeks of mindfulness meditation can decrease grey matter density in the amygdala, for instance, which could make an expert meditator less easily frightened (by a lion surprising them on a savanna, say, or their boss demanding, "I want to see you in my office, now!").

Another brain region commonly affected by meditation is the insula—the reward-related brain area that makes us enjoy helping others. And then there is the hippocampus, which has nothing to do with camps for hippo-lovers and everything to do with emotions and memory. Atrophy of this horseshoe-shaped area (hence the "hippo," which comes from Greek *hippos*, meaning "horse") has also been linked with Alzheimer's disease. A typical meditation expert, meanwhile, will have a particularly large hippocampus compared to an average Joe, suggesting possible protection against dementia and Alzheimer's disease. Such an increased volume of the hippocampus resulting from meditation has been explained by hikes in the levels of a protein called BDNF—brain-derived neurotrophic factor—which helps the development and survival of nerve cells in the brain.

Spikes in BDNF are one of the reasons why physical exercise is good for your brain. On the other hand, stress makes the levels of blood BDNF wane. That's bad news. A person whose body runs low on BDNF is at a higher risk for Parkinson's disease, Alzheimer's disease, multiple sclerosis, and even suicide. Post-mortem tests on the brains of suicide victims reveal that they tend to have decreased levels of this protein. Suicide apart, BDNF seems to predict mortality all on its own, at least in women. Eighty-five-year-old Danes who have the lowest levels of BDNF in their blood plasma have over twice the risk of death as do women with the highest levels. Now, if you want to raise your blood levels of BDNF, go for a downward-facing dog pose and start meditating. Volunteers participating in a three-month yoga and meditation retreat saw their plasma levels of BDNF triple, while a shorter twelve-week intervention caused a two-fold increase in BDNF.

Another thing you may find changed in the blood of people who meditate are their leukocytes—the white blood cells involved in the functioning of the immune system. To see if I could nudge my own leukocytes with a bit of mindfulness, I visited the London offices of a biotech company called Oxford MediStress, a spinoff of the University of Oxford.

The interior of the building I entered, just off Tottenham Court Road, looked somewhere in between sleek and start-up-y. David Sarphie, who holds a PhD in biomedical engineering from the University of Oxford and who co-founded Oxford MediStress, led me into a white corporate kitchen, where he had already prepared the tools he would use to evaluate the responsiveness of my immune system. As we settled around a long, glossy table, he explained to me the workings of the measure they'd developed, called leukocyte coping capacity (LCC). When you get stressed, Sarphie told me, your leukocytes start producing reactive oxygen species, the very same molecules that are implicated in cellular damage and aging. To evaluate their levels, you take a drop of blood and mix it with a chemical called phorbol myristate acetate. "It kind of pokes the white blood cells and says, 'respond, respond,'" Sarphie explained. This way you can see the levels of reactive oxygen species your leukocytes are spewing out. The more reactive oxygen species, the lower your LCC score will be (which is generally bad).

This reactivity of leukocytes had already been used in several studies to measure stress in creatures as diverse as wild badgers and young humans. When a group of students watched the 1974 version of *The Texas Chainsaw Massacre*, their leukocytes fired out tons of reactive oxygen species, and their LCC scores plummeted, suggesting that their immune systems got temporarily messed up by the stress. So if you ever find yourself affected by a bacterial infection, don't indulge in a horror-movie marathon at that very moment—instead of helping you feel better, it could make your immune system less efficient.

As we chatted about sore throats and chainsaw murderers, Sarphie started preparing a test kit for the day's experiment. It would involve just one subject: me. First was the unpleasant part. With a tool that resembles an icing syringe, Sarphie poked the tip of my index finger to get a few drops of my blood. Then he plopped the sample into an "incubator," which to me looked like an old-school answering machine. And then, we waited. After ten minutes, Sarphie showed me my initial results, which, I have to admit, I found slightly disappointing. My LCC scores were okay, but not as high as I'd imagined (I had secretly hoped that my leukocytes were these black-belt infection-fighting masters—they were not).

The second part of our little "experiment" involved me sitting in the lotus position for about half an hour and practising mindfulness meditation. That part was fun. I found a secluded terrace overlooking the back gardens of London, positioned myself in a sunny spot far from prying eyes, and off I went. I moved my attention inward. I observed my body, my mind. I noticed my breath flowing in and out, in and out. And then I started thinking about the flea collars I should buy for my dogs. Argh. I moved my attention back to my breath. In, out, in, out. I started thinking about rearranging shelves in my daughter's bedroom. I inhaled and brought my attention once again back to the present moment. The flea collars popped up. Inhale, exhale. And so it continued.

After my mindfulness session, I went back to see Sarphie. He tortured my index finger some more and placed the new blood sample in the incubator. Ten minutes later we had the results, and my LCC scores had gone up! Okay, maybe they didn't exactly skyrocket, more like inched up, but we could definitely see some improvement. A single session of mindfulness shifted my leukocytes toward a more healthy behaviour of firing out less reactive oxygen species.

Although I didn't manage to get a large response from my own immune system, it's hardly surprising—I'm a Sunday meditator at best (hence the thoughts of flea collars and shelves). Studies done on people who have far more experience in meditation and practise more regularly show better results. Take the one done at the University of Wisconsin-Madison that involved sixty-eight volunteers. About half of them were meditation pros, each with an average of nine thousand lifetime hours of chanting and attention-focusing under the belt. The other half of the group was made up of people of similar age who were not into mind-body practices. After some initial medical tests and psychological evaluations, the researchers applied a rather nasty concoction to the volunteers' forearms—a cream containing capsaicin, the same compound that makes chili peppers burn your mouth. Right afterward, it was stress time. The volunteers had to do a five-minute impromptu speech and some mental arithmetic in front of two stern-looking judges and a video camera—something that most people find quite anxiety-inducing. Then it was back to prodding and poking, as well as measuring the extent of the inflammatory reaction to the capsaicin on their forearms.

Later on, when the researchers analyzed the results, they discovered that the experienced meditators had less cortisol in their saliva after the upsetting speech experience, and that the red, inflamed areas on their arms was on average much smaller, too, suggesting that their immune systems were less "jumpy." Which makes me wonder: if a mindfulness expert fell into a patch of poison ivy, would they break out in a less severe rash than I would in such a scenario? And no, I'm not willing to check.

Poison ivy and various unpleasant creatures were certainly a risk to those of our ancestors who were ostracized from their tribes and left to wander in nature all alone. Remember how they developed increased inflammation (to protect them from bacteria in wounds) and lowered antiviral protection (not much needed since they were away from their snotty peers)? This so-called conserved transcriptional response to adversity is no longer beneficial to us in the modern world, yet it is quite widespread due to chronic stress. It also tends to lead to diabetes, rheumatoid arthritis, and strokes.

Fortunately, though, meditation may reverse these processes. The positive effects of meditation reach down all the way to the DNA level—even after just a few weeks of meditation, you can see reduced expression of pro-inflammatory genes in white blood cells. Genes associated with antiviral protection, on the other hand, get upregulated (their expression is increased). Think of it as playing with the volume knob on the radio: when you meditate, the level of inflammation goes down, while the power of your virus-fighting squads goes up. So here is a tip: try meditation before your next round of vaccinations. Experiments with the flu vaccine confirm that this can help produce higher antibody titres, lowering the chances of you ending up sick despite the injection. Unfortunately, fifteen minutes of Zen in the doctor's office while you await your inoculations won't do the trick. You need to practise for at least a few weeks ahead of time.

In case vaccinations make you think of needles, and needles make you think of pain, what a short meditation session could help you with is the level of prick-induced suffering you might experience. In one experiment, volunteers had to rate how much it hurt them when researchers applied a pad heated to 120 degrees Fahrenheit (49°C) to their leg—about as scorching as the water from a hot water tap. The study participants, who had no prior experience with meditation, were randomly divided into groups: some were instructed to meditate as their limbs were being semi-tortured, while others read excerpts from an eighteenth-century publication with a high boredom potential called *The Natural History and Antiquities of Selborne*. The results showed that a short session of mindfulness meditation reduced the perception of pain by 27 percent compared to the experience of a control group who received no special instructions. The book, meanwhile, made it about 14 percent worse. The benefits of meditation were not exclusively due to a placebo effect, either. Some volunteers had a sham analgesic cream applied to their legs before the pad was put in use, and their pain ratings were lower by only 11 percent—better than the book but not as good as meditation.

Some experiments suggest that meditation can work on pain in a similar fashion to ibuprofen (although the magnitude of the effect is still mostly unknown). When people with lots of meditation experience go for an intense one-day retreat, you can see changes in the expression of their *COX2* gene. Aspirin and ibuprofen also work to dull aches because they target *COX2*, putting brakes on the pain-promoting enzymes it helps churn out.

Admittedly, there is still not enough evidence to claim that all meditation is a miracle drug. For now, the authors of a 2016 review published in the prestigious *Annals of the New York Academy of Sciences* caution against "exaggerating the positive effects" of meditation on the immune system. Something is obviously there, but how much exactly, we don't yet know. As scientists love to say, "more research is needed."

The type of meditation that has been the most studied so far is mindfulness meditation. That's the very thing that is so in vogue all over the internet, from Pinterest to gossip columns on the lives of California celebrities. And no, it's not the same as mindfulness. Mindfulness is simply being aware of the present moment, whether it's smelling the roses or listening to the sound of running water as you do the dishes.

Mindfulness meditation, by contrast, is a practice that takes time and commitment, and which helps you become more mindful in your everyday life. Much of the research is based on something even more precise, mindfulness-based stress reduction, an eight-week program developed back in the 1970s by Jon Kabat-Zinn, professor of medicine at the University of Massachusetts Medical School. These days the name Kabat-Zinn and mindfulness are utterly linked (take any decent book on mindfulness and chances are, Kabat-Zinn wrote the introduction). The program itself involves intensive training in mindfulness meditation, with its key ingredients being acceptance and lack of judgement. Kabat-Zinn says our thoughts are like a waterfall, and mindfulness is like finding a cave behind the cascade: "We still see and hear the water, but we are out of the torrent."

While practising mindfulness meditation, you are not supposed to force your mind into blankness. When your thoughts wander, and they almost always do—to your shopping list or your unanswered emails—you don't judge yourself; you don't say, "I'm terrible at meditation." Instead you just try to return to the present moment, to observing sensations in your body. You don't strive to change these sensations, either. If your left toe hurts, you don't try to diminish the pain. You accept it.

Besides many promising direct links between mindfulness training and health, MSBR and related programs may influence our lifespans and physical wellness in a circular way. Mindfulness makes people ruminate less. It boosts empathy. Weirdly enough, mindfulness meditation can also push people to eat more veggies and fruits—and it's not just that the yoga types usually love kale smoothies anyway, since randomized trials show these effects, too. The explanation may lie in the way practising mindful attention helps people fight cravings. Instead of just following that hollow feeling in your mouth prompting you to reach for a cookie, you acknowledge it, observe it, and let it go—and then you reach for an apple instead.

In a similar fashion, mindfulness has been shown to quench cravings for cigarettes, a finding confirmed by neuroimaging studies. When smokers who practise meditation look at images of people puffing tobacco, craving-related areas of their brains don't light up as much as they do in other nicotine addicts. For each day per week of meditation practice, smokers light up 1.52 fewer cigarettes. This may not seem like much, but when you consider that a single cigarette shortens lifespan by eleven minutes, daily meditation may add about two hours of life each and every week. As a bonus, these mindfulness-sponsored extra days may also prove to be more pleasant—that's because mindfulness-based stress reduction programs help alleviate feelings of loneliness. Romantic couples may thrive on these programs as well. The more mindful one partner is, the less likely they are to act in an overly negative or aggressive way during conflicts, and they will also be more forgiving.

One thing that's particularly damaging to relationships is what psychologists refer to as "stress spillover." Imagine you had a bad day at work. Your boss was unfair, your colleagues were annoying, your projects fell through. You come home grumpy. The moment you cross the threshold, your partner starts throwing some minor household grievance at you (perhaps the car needs to be fixed). You feel your emotions boiling, and you explode. A nasty fight follows. Mindfulness interventions, meanwhile, make people more aware of their feelings and more collected in their responses—instead of blowing up at your partner about the car, you might just say that you are upset after work and need time to yourself. The fight is averted.

Another mechanism through which mindfulness-based stress reduction may improve relationships is related to the key ingredients of mindfulness: non-judgement and acceptance. By honing acceptance skills during meditation, partners may become more tolerant of their loved ones' shortcomings and imperfections. Instead of dwelling on the dirty socks left in the middle of the room, you just breathe deeply and let it go. Studies confirm that greater levels of mindfulness correlate to greater satisfaction in romantic relationships. Randomized experiments take it even further, showing that eight-week-long mindfulness programs can increase relationship satisfaction. Now consider that a good marriage can reduce mortality by a staggering 49 percent (to a healthy diet's 26 percent or so), and you see why mindfulness in relationships could also be good for your centenarian potential.

There is one caveat, however. Some psychologists suggest that meditation may work only for committed relationships—no matter if they are experiencing temporary troubles or just want to add to their happiness. If a couple is not really into staying together in the first place, enhanced mindfulness could backfire. Imagine Mr. A, who for a few years now has been in an informal relationship with Ms. B. Mr. A is not exactly happy with how the whole thing is going, but he also can't pinpoint what's wrong. In truth, he doesn't give the relationship much thought at all. They fight, they make up, life goes on. Then, one day, Mr. A signs up for a mindfulness course. After a couple of weeks he becomes more mindful of his own thoughts and feelings. He starts to notice how his stomach clenches every time Ms. B comes home from work. He picks up on more negative undertones in her comments. He realizes he is no longer happy. He decides to leave.

Assuming lack of commitment is not an issue, one type of meditation that is often recommended for couples is something called "loving-kindness." It may sound New Agey, but the effects of this practice can be seen in brain activation patterns and in DNA changes. Loving-kindness involves thinking compassionate thoughts directed at other people, like, "may XY be happy," "may XY be healthy," and so on. The exercise is repeated by placing different individuals as the XY, from your loved ones and acquaintances (your mail carrier), to strangers (the old lady on the bus), and then to people you actually dislike (your unfair boss). Such training has been shown to change brain activation in areas responsible for empathy and pain perception.

While research on direct physical effects of loving-kindness is still meagre, evidence of its potential role as a tool for increasing social connectedness is more convincing. This particular type of intervention not only increases empathy but also makes people less biased and simply nicer. A common theme reported by participants after loving-kindness trainings are changes in their relationships. One professional woman who used to easily lose her temper with her elderly mother confessed, "When I enter her room now, I can feel myself soften." After two weeks of loving-kindness meditation, people are willing to donate almost twice as much money as are those assigned to other personality development interventions. This hike in charity also coincides with changes in brain responses to suffering. And since empathy, charity donations, and social connections are all important for longevity, these findings are likely not trivial.

What may be more questionable in terms of health effects is an intervention that is often sold alongside loving-kindness: gratitude journalling. In fact, it may be quite oversold. Take a look at the shelves of any large bookstore and you will see plenty of publications touting life-changing results of gratitude, like *Living in Gratitude: A Journey that Will Change Your Life,* or *Grateful: The Transformative Power of Giving Thanks.* Handy gratitude journals, with space to scribble down your thoughts each day, promise to make giving thanks easier and aesthetically pleasant—even glitter is possible if you are into stuff like that. In your journal or in your head, you are supposed to count your blessings. Write or think what you are grateful for: for being healthy, for having a warm house, for having enough food not to go hungry, for sunshine and birds, for smooth driving on the Cross Bronx Expressway (which supposedly borders on a miracle).

You can also compose a thank-you letter to someone who was nice to you or even pay them a "gratitude visit." Just to make it clear: gratitude is not a type of meditation. It's supposed to work through fostering positive emotions while quelling stress and worry. But the evidence on the physiological effects of gratitude is mixed. Most of the self-help literature appears to be based on a few studies conducted by the same team of researchers back in 2003. They did indeed conclude that students who, for two and a half months, wrote down five things per week they could be thankful for, be it "waking up this morning" or "the Rolling Stones" (a real example), experienced fewer symptoms of physical illness as a result. Later on a number of experiments reported better sleep, fewer headaches, and lower levels of inflammatory biomarkers in grateful people, but many other trials showed no effects of gratitude on health. A 2017 review of thirty-eight studies concluded that "those expecting huge and lasting gains, or 'life-changing' outcomes from the activity, are likely to be disappointed."

Don't get me wrong: I'm not saying not to do it. If you enjoy it, practising gratitude certainly won't hurt you. It will quite likely make you a nicer person, and it may even improve your health. Yet if your time or your mental resources are limited, there are things you can try for "life-changing outcomes" that have stronger scientific evidence behind them—like mindful meditation or yoga.

The Colour of Pain

One of my husband's work colleagues, Thorbjørn Knudsen, besides being an outstanding academic researcher, is also a skilful yogi. So skilful in fact that he was a subject of studies conducted in Germany on mind-body connections.

Knudsen looks as unlike the Maharishi Mahesh Yogi–standard as possible: when I talk with him he is dressed in a white collared shirt and dark jeans. He is clean-shaven, with short, neat hair and understated glasses. Very business school prof, very not yogi. Yet Knudsen is a living proof that you don't need flowing robes and sandals to impress others with your yoga skills. He certainly did leave a lasting impression on the researchers at the University Hospital of Cologne—one of the largest medical institutions in Germany. For the experiments there Knudsen engaged in a practice called Nadi Shodhana, which is Sanskrit for "channel purification." It involves breathing through alternate nostrils: in through the left one, out through the right, in and out, as slowly as possible.

He was seated in a bland research room, covered in a flowered orange blanket to keep warm, while his head was plastered all over with electrodes for measuring brain activity. As he did his Nadi Shodhana, the scientists also measured Knudsen's heart rate and his blood pressure, which he was supposed to try lower. To get precise results, they asked to put a catheter through the blood vessels in his arms all the way to his heart. Knudsen was unexcited about the whole catheter idea: "Part of the yoga training was how to deal with pain, but still I was like, 'Hmmm . . . Okay,'" he says.

Once he agreed to the procedure and the catheter went in, the measurements began. Knudsen kept breathing. Left nostril. Right nostril. Slow, slow, very slow. Suddenly, a commotion in the lab caught his attention. "There was this one guy observing it from the outside, and he storms in and shouts 'Stop! Stop!'" he recalls. Knudsen had managed to lower his blood pressure to an astoundingly low 40 over 20, causing the scientists to panic. They were worried he was close to death or at least to passing out. But Knudsen was surprised by the whole fuss. He was perfectly fine—just doing his yoga. The researchers admitted to him after the experiment that they'd never seen such blood pressure–lowering ability before.

In another trial at the same lab, Knudsen's body was assaulted with extreme noise, with needles, and with a bucketful of ice, all to check whether there would be any disturbance in his brainwaves as he meditated. There wasn't. Nothing could break the calm pattern of his brain activity.

In everyday life, Knudsen sometimes likes to play with his mind-body abilities. "At some point I wanted to see how far I could go," he says. He had a tooth in need of a root canal, so he asked his dentist to do the procedure without anaesthesia. To deal with the pain, Knudsen used a yoga practice called pratyahara, which means literally "gaining mastery over external influences." First, you meditate to relax. Then, in that relaxed state, "you treat the pain as a person that's very interesting to you," Knudsen says. "It has a colour, it has a sound, it has a smell, taste. You do not force the mind to stop thinking of the pain. On the contrary, you let your mind fully experience that pain while, at the same time, you observe your mind. At some point, the mind loses interest in the pain in the same way you may lose interest in some annoying person who is sitting next to you on the plane." Although, he admits that the pain of the root canal treatment was challenging, pratyahara made it manageable.

Already as many as one in twenty-five Americans and one in twenty-six Canadians practise yoga, and half a million Britons do so regularly, yet for most it certainly doesn't mean pratyahara or alternate nostril breathing. They are also unlikely to be capable of managing root canal pain with their skills. In all probability, though, their health does profit from all the yoga they do—and, according to one review of studies, potentially more so than if they simply replaced their practice with some other form of exercise, like walking or stretching. The review concluded that "yoga interventions appear to be equal or superior to exercise in nearly every outcome measured except those involving physical fitness." So if your goal is to complete an Ironman triathlon, then yoga is not necessarily for you, but if you want to simply stay healthy, go for it. Yoga may be good for the management of diabetes and the boosting of the immune system; and, for patients with fibromyalgia, yoga can bring greater relief of symptoms than FDA-recommended drug therapies.

Yoga might be particularly beneficial for heart rate variability—that easily measurable indicator of the proper functioning of your fight-and-flight response. A curious series of experiments involving albino rats showed that if you teach the animals something resembling yoga breathing, they'll become more stress-resistant. Training rats in the rodent equivalent of pranayama, breath-control yoga, doesn't involve sitting on exercise mats around a Maharishi Mahesh Yogi look-alike and sipping organic matcha. It involves conditioning them in a piece of lab equipment with a rather evil-sounding name, a "plethysmography chamber," which resembles a small Plexiglas space rocket for rats. If you place an animal inside that space rocket, it will measure the creature's respiratory rate, which is basically the number of inhalations and exhalations it does per minute.

To practise control over their respiratory rate, the rodents were trained with unpleasant stroboscopic LED lights that flooded their plethysmography chambers from above and below. The glare would turn off only if the animal managed to slow down its breathing to eighty breaths per minute or less. A control group of rodents, meanwhile, had to endure the lights turning on and off haphazardly, no matter what they did. Such two-hour sessions went on for a month, five times per week (life's not easy when you are a lab rat).

Once the researchers confirmed that the "yoga rats" did start breathing more slowly as a default, it was time for some extra stress for the animals. One such classic test entails letting the rodents out into a large arena. This may sound like a reprieve after the confines of plethysmography chambers, but for rats it's not necessarily fun—a wide, open space brings to mind soaring hawks and other dangers swooping from the air. That's why the more a rodent is stressed, the more time it will spend hugging the walls instead of exploring the centre. Here is where the difference between the yoga rats and the rest showed up: while the control animals spent on average seventy seconds cowering away from the scary vastness, the rodents trained in slow breathing started exploring after less than half that time. In another stress test, once more involving equipment with a wicked name ("rodent restrainer"), the rats were held in claustrophobic cylindrical tubes for ten minutes. And once again the yoga rats proved less stressed by the experience.

Remarkably, it's not just chilled-out rats that breathe more slowly—mindful people do so, too. While at rest, long-term practitioners of mindful meditation inhale and exhale fewer times per minute than your typical human. They also blink less and in a different pattern. Look at an average person and you will see that their eyelids go up and down quite erratically: sometimes they'll blink in a rapid succession, other times they will stare at you as if playing the who-will-blink-first game. Long-term meditators, on the other hand, have a very regular blinking pattern, and a much slower one at that. These slow-breathing, slow-blinking meditators are not just a curiosity. Spontaneous eye blink rate is a reflection of how the dopamine system works in your brain (abnormal blinking is a sign of Parkinson's disease, for example). Fast breathing, meanwhile, can signify anxiety.

By now you may be wondering what it takes to become a "long-term meditator." In the eye-blinking study, it meant a minimum of 1,439 hours of meditation experience. In the respiration rate study, it was at least three years with daily routines of thirty minutes or more. This may seem daunting, but the truth is that with meditation and yoga the more you practise, the more benefits you will likely reap. It doesn't necessarily mean that if you can't commit to a daily half-hour of practice for years on end you should just throw in the towel and go shopping for goji berries instead. Short bursts of mind-body exercises work too—just less well. Even though the activity of the enzyme that protects the tips of chromosomes, telomerase, can increase after just a few weeks of mindfulness-based stress reduction, it may take as long as a year to see the results in telomere length. In a similar vein, the effects of mindfulness meditation on the immune system seem dosage-dependent, too: the longer you do it the more your anti-infection troops profit, and the more your inflammatory markers decrease.

But don't rush just yet to squeeze pratyahara into every spare minute you have. Doing yoga while cooking dinner or brushing your kids' teeth won't necessarily do you that much good. The quality of your engagement counts as well. Kabat-Zinn once wrote, "Five minutes of formal practice can be as profound or more so than forty-five minutes . . . the sincerity of your effort matters far more than elapsed time." What does it mean to practise "well"? In mindfulness, it means attempting to return to present-moment experience, no matter how pleasant or unpleasant it may be. It means telling yourself that "It's okay to experience this." It means trying to feel all sensations in your body, including the lousy ones (itchy noses, hurting knees). It means that you don't zone out completely or doze off on your couch.

Of course, the more you practise, the more the quality of your meditation or yoga tends to improve as well. One good way to give yourself a quick mind-body experience boost is to sign up for a retreat. Choices abound—from Zen meditation gardens in Arizona and asana classes in the forests of Bhutan to ten-day Vipassana courses taught in over 165 centres around the world. For cold lovers, there are even snow-yoga retreats in the Alps. The good news is that it doesn't have to be expensive—the Vipassana meditation retreats are free of charge (sponsored by voluntary donations from previous students). No matter what you choose, studies show that meditation and yoga retreats tend to be particularly helpful, and it's not simply because they make for a relaxing holiday—the "retreat effect" goes beyond "vacation effect."

Now, in terms of what practice you should pick, the jury is still out. In some scientific reviews, all meditation and yoga styles come out as interchangeable. One such comparison based on over three hundred trials, which included an astounding fifty-three yoga types (there really are that many), found that all brought similar health benefits. On the other hand, neuroimaging studies report that different meditation techniques activate and deactivate different parts of the brain. A few hints exist as well that for preventing some illnesses, some practices could be more effective than others. If you want to reduce your risk of cardiovascular disease, for instance, transcendental meditation may be a particularly good idea.

Apart from that, many researchers agree that at this point the best option is to simply choose the practice that you find the most appealing. It may be mindfulness meditation, hatha yoga, tai chi or even qigong—ancient Chinese exercises that are supposed to balance the flow of qi through the body. Whether you believe in harmonious movements of energy or not, both tai chi and qigong have the potential to bring health benefits: tai chi has been linked to the reduction of severity of fibromyalgia, while qigong may help with fatigue and boost the activity of telomerase. Admittedly, however, research on tai chi and qigong is quite limited, and we still have absolutely no idea if any of these practices can actually prolong life.

⧖

Long-term meditators reap some very real profits from their practices—from longer telomeres to improved immune systems. Does that mean we should all be getting "prescription meditation" from our doctors? It's too early to tell. Certainly there are promising indications that even short-term engagements in yoga or mindfulness could boost the levels of neuron-growing proteins in your blood, make pain less painful, and possibly even slow down your epigenetic clocks. Yet the evidence for the life-extending powers of meditation doesn't seem as strong as that for marriage or for fighting loneliness. We also don't really know how the effects of yoga or mindfulness-based stress reduction might compare to those of other interventions such as exercise and super-healthy nutrition. On the other hand, the research that we already do have suggests that just a few minutes of mind-body practice a day could make it easier for you to achieve all your other longevity goals: it could improve your romantic relationship, help rid you of loneliness, or ease nicotine cravings. Since most studies on the health effects of mindfulness or yoga control for diets, exercise, smoking, and so on, the benefits of such practices could be underestimated (a mindfulness buff might be eating lots of vegetables precisely because they picked up mindfulness in the first place).

What's more, meditating or doing a few yoga asanas is cheap and easy. There is no need to rush to a gym or buy any special gadgets. No need to buy anything, in fact: just find a quiet spot and relax. Feel your breath. Let your brain rewire. Even if some Pinterest-based promises of what mind-body routines can do for you are exaggerated—certainly your life is unlikely to get completely, miraculously transformed—your health will benefit and so will your mind. You may become calmer, more focused, emotionally stronger. You may grow—and not just younger.

A FEW SUGGESTIONS TO BOOST YOUR LONGEVITY

Choose the mind-body technique you find the most appealing, be it yoga, mindfulness, or tai chi, and try to practise regularly and long-term: the more you stick with it the more benefits you will get. If you are striving to change other health-related things in your life—to eat more veggies, stop smoking, stop fighting with your spouse—meditation can make it easier, too. If you want a quick boost, sign up for a retreat. And don't watch horror movies if you are down with a virus: it could make your immune system less efficient. Try mindfulness or a few asanas instead.

LONGEVITY LESSONS
FROM JAPAN

Ikigai, Cherry Blossoms, and Working Till You Drop

IT'S A GREY, DRIZZLY AFTERNOON in the Greater Tokyo area, yet seventy-year-old Fujita Masatoshi seems undisturbed by the weather. Clad in blue overalls, he is busy at work at his post-retirement employment—clipping trees around the parking lot of the Silver Human Resources Center in Matsudo City. The pay is poor, but Masatoshi says money is not an issue. After years behind a desk at a transportation company, he has more than enough saved up for a lazy retirement. But lazy isn't something that Masatoshi is after. He may like tennis and baseball, but, he says, "that isn't enough." What he needs is *ikigai*, purpose in life, and that's why one day at the age of sixty-five he showed up at the Silver Human Resources Center and asked for employment—joining 49 percent of Japanese men this age who work at silver-hair jobs.

Search for a book on longevity and, chances are, you will come across something with "Japan" in the title. There is a good reason for that. At the time of writing, Japan held the title of the longest-living nation on earth, with their record life expectancy at birth at 84.2 years. That's almost six years longer than the average American can expect to live, a year and a half longer than a Canadian, and almost three years longer than a Briton. Japan also tops the charts with the highest number of centenarians per capita, and while I was travelling across Japan researching this book, the oldest person in the world, a Japanese woman, died there at the age of 117—older than the country of Australia.

Yet Japan hasn't always been a longevity paradise. Right after World War Two, an average Japanese man could expect to live a mere fifty years, and a woman fifty-four years. By 1986, however, the country had already climbed to the top of the world for female life expectancy. What happened? Before the twentieth century, hunger was the norm, and only the rapid post-war economic growth made malnutrition a thing of the past for most. Moreover, as the country developed, the health care system received a tremendous boost. Now basically everyone had medical insurance and was guaranteed regular checkups. Mortality rates for communicable diseases such as tuberculosis plummeted, extending average lifespans.

If you've ever had sushi or miso soup for dinner and felt the next day as if your body had doubled in size overnight, you've experienced the dark side of the Japanese diet—its saltiness (the post-sushi puffiness is the result of water retention). Back in the 1950s, a typical Yamada Tarō and Yamada Hanako, the Japanese equivalent Mr. and Ms. Smith, ate on average thirty grams of table salt per day—that's a staggeringly high number compared to the current USDA recommendations of less than six grams. Almost everything savoury, it seemed, contained salt: soy sauce, tsukemono pickles, ramen noodles, miso soup. As a result, high blood pressure and strokes were ubiquitous. It was in large part due to public awareness campaigns that the diet has shifted away from such high sodium levels, and average lifespan lengthened. Yet even today, at ten grams per day, the Japanese still eat quite a lot of salt.

All that blood pressure–raising sodium notwithstanding, the Japanese diet is certainly one of the main reasons for the country's remarkable longevity. It's based on high consumption of seafood, vegetables, seaweed, and soy, with minimal dairy or meat. What's more, the Japanese have a saying, *hara hachi bu*—eat only until you are 80 percent full. From a research perspective, it makes perfect sense. Experiments on many animal species show that calorie restriction can prolong life—suggesting it might also work in humans.

This unsurprising advice coming from Japan—don't stuff yourself, eat more vegetables and less meat—has inspired some people to look for more wonder-like Japanese foods that could add years of life without too much effort. Some have said it's horse meat. Others have suggested ginger. Yet others have pointed to resveratrol, the polyphenol found in grapes, which are particularly popular in Japan's longest-living prefecture, Nagano. If dining on horse meat stewed in ginger and grape sauce sounds like a disturbing longevity-boosting idea, rest assured: just like with many other miracle foods, from turmeric to moringa, there is not much science to support it.

In general, Japanese people are obsessed with health—although their obsession may be of a different sort than the North American one. In Japan it's far less about gluten-free eating and miracle foods and more about blood tests and colonoscopy (although I myself would take goji berries over intestinal exams any day). Across the country, about three million people each year undergo what is called there the "human dry dock" screening. They check into hospitals for at least a day and submit themselves to a whole series of tests, such as chest X-rays, weight measurements, blood tests, urine tests, radiography, and yes, colonoscopy. Among Japanese men age forty-five to fifty-four, over 70 percent have some form of checkup at least once per year.

Admittedly, Japanese people have been obsessed with health and hygiene long before colonoscopy tubes were invented. Valuing purity is a tradition in Shinto, where evil is associated with all things dirty. Already in the third century, Chinese historians were commenting on the extraordinary cleanliness of the Japanese—now imagine how the locals must have perceived the stinky Europeans who began arriving in the sixteenth century.

Although focus on hygiene certainly does play a role in Japanese longevity, some researchers have also looked for answers in the DNA of the local population. We are talking about an island nation, after all, one that was basically closed off to the world for centuries. Maybe people here evolved some special mutation that allows them to have these extra years of life? Indeed, there may be something to this line of thinking. Take a gene called *ApoE*, of which one particular allele, *ApoE4*, is rarely found among the Japanese. Carriers of the *ApoE4* allele, many of whom are of Scandinavian descent, are at about 40 percent higher risk of heart disease than those with variants of the gene that are more common in Japan. And then there are the *FOXO* genes, implicated in longevity of hydras, whales, and Jeanne Calment—and American men of Japanese ancestry.

Another genetic variation that may be helping the average Yamada Tarō and Yamada Hanako live long is something that's easy to spot the moment you set foot in Japan. For me, the realization hit me over the head, literally, when I banged my forehead on a regular door frame for the first time in my life. As a five-foot-six-inch (168 cm) woman living in Europe, I'm used to being on the short side of society. Not in Japan. Suddenly, I could reach top shelves in the kitchen of my Airbnb rental and had to mind low-hanging lamps. I was about four inches (10 cm) taller than average! Meanwhile, studies suggest that being short is good for longevity (which could also help explain why men on average die earlier than women). For example, generally shortish Greeks and Italians who move to Australia tend to outlive the taller locals by about four years. So here is a tip: if you are a young woman and you want your future kids to live to a hundred, don't go for the super-tall guys—pick the Tom Cruises of the world instead.

Yet although the height and meat-eating ApoE genes may be playing for Japanese longevity, other genes are playing against them.

The Japanese are, for example, more genetically susceptible to developing diabetes and becoming overweight (although you wouldn't know it from checking out people on the streets—only 2.2 percent of Japanese men and 3.5 percent of Japanese women are obese). One way or the other, genetics contribute only in part to the overall good health of the inhabitants of Nippon. When the Japanese relocate to California, rates of heart disease among them double.

Diet, genetics, dry dock checkups, and hygiene are all surely important factors in Japanese longevity. But they are not the whole story—far from it. There is a saying in the land of cherry blossoms: *yamai wa ki kara*—"sickness and health start with the mind." Research shows it does indeed, and that no amount of miracle foods can replace social cohesion or having ikigai.

The Longevity Village

I pulled my car over into the tiny parking spot by the narrow ribbon of the Kohachiga River, tucked in between the lush bumps of the lower Japanese Alps. The day was cloudy, the air moist and smelling of greenery. I took a few steps toward rocks marked with characters I couldn't decipher. Out of one mossy stone, water gushed, disappearing through a rather unappealing metal grate below. But this was not just any water—according to a local legend, it's longevity water. It seemed that with the help of Google Maps, I had found the elixir of life. If only Ponce de Léon had been there.

I reached for a cup that had been conveniently left nearby and poured myself some of the water. I took a gulp, waiting for magic to happen. Nothing happened. Unless, that is, some local waterborne bug was already installing itself in my stomach, preparing for an assault. Yet I was certainly no younger and didn't feel any renewed energy. I put the cup away and got back into the car. I was on my way to see more convincing reasons than miracle water for the outstanding longevity of people who live among the peaks of the Japanese Alps.

The Nagano prefecture, famed across the world for the Winter Olympics of 1998, has in recent years overtaken Okinawa as the Japanese epicenter of longevity. While in the early 2000s there were many publications with the words "Okinawa" and "Diet" in their titles, you might soon start seeing books about the "Nagano Diet." Without doubt, diet is part of Nagano's success. Because the area is mountainous, it was hard to grow rice here, and because it's away from the coast, seafood wasn't easily available. Instead, the locals ate plenty of vegetables and soy. Today, the people of Nagano still top the nation's charts when it comes to vegetable consumption—they down 27 percent more greens than does an average Yamada Tarō.

Yet as I arrived at the small village of Matsukawa in the Nagano prefecture, this love of vegetables was certainly not apparent. I'm not sure what I was expecting, really. Perhaps roadside stalls selling heads of fresh-from-the farm cabbage and lettuce? Small yet busy markets where locals mill around buying celery stalks, turnips, and enoki mushrooms? I saw nothing of that. Instead there were several big-box stores offering plastic-wrapped vegetables not much different from those at any supermarket in the West. Oh, well. My romantic vision of a veggie-loving countryside shattered, I continued deeper into the village. And there I did see something that gave me an insight into Matsukawa's longevity secret: commitment to the community.

From all the Nagano's mountain villages, I chose to visit the unassuming Matsukawa for a reason: this is the place where men live the longest in the whole of Japan—82.2 years on average, over ten years longer than the male inhabitants of Mississippi. Their longevity formula does include the veggie-loaded diet, but researchers studying the remarkable health of the locals point to two other key factors: social cohesion and the commitment to community.

I could certainly see this the moment I arrived at a park in the centre of Matsukawa. First of all, the area was spotless. Not a single piece of trash was visible, and nothing was out of place or broken—no spatial stigma risk here for sure. The facilities were impressive and designed for all. There was a playground, a picnic site, outdoor fitness equipment for adults, a public library, a stage for events, a foot-massage path (you take off your shoes and walk over various types of spikes—painful; I've tried). The toilets were so sparklingly clean my grandma would have been proud, and she is the Martha Stewart of cleaning. There were even fresh flowers beside the sinks. You could see that this was a place where some very conscientious people truly cared about where they lived. As I strolled around, kindergarten-age children ran alone across the park with no helicopter parents in sight. Two old ladies chatted in the picnic area while another one biked to the library. It was not the picture of communal hustle and bustle you can witness in Latin countries, but everything was orderly and smooth-running. It was an image of a collectivist nation at work.

Before the second half of the twentieth century, there wasn't much talk about collectivist or individualistic cultures. But then, in the 1970s, Geert Hofstede, a Dutch employee of IBM who later became a professor of social psychology, came across a large survey database of IBM workers in over fifty countries, containing more than a hundred thousand questionnaires. On a hunch, Hofstede started analyzing the data and discovered it to be an amazing treasure trove of cross-country comparisons. This set him on a long journey of studying contrasts between cultures. Today, Hofstede's cultural dimensions model is widely used to examine how people across the planet differ in their approach to life.

One of Hofstede's dimensions is collectivism-individualism. Citizens of countries that score high on individualism tend to have an "I" mentality, and you hear them talk a lot about things such as privacy, individual rights, and achievement. A large, tightly knit family to depend on is not part of the picture. As De Tocqueville once said, "Such folk owe no man anything and hardly expect anything from anybody." In a collectivist nation, the focus is on the group—the priority here is harmony and belonging. Loyalty is treasured, and decisions are based on what's best for everyone. This type of culture is a "we" culture.

As you may have suspected, the US is a very individualistic nation. In Hofstede's calculations, it came out as number one in the world with a score of 91 (on a scale of 0 to 100). The UK got 89; Canada, 80; France, 71; Poland, 60; and Japan scored 46, which placed it on the collectivistic end of the spectrum, although still quite far from the most collectivistic country of all, Guatemala—a mere 6. In Guatemala, family is extremely important. Many people live in the same house with their extended family—cousins, aunts, and uncles included—and when they emigrate to the US, they take their relatives with them (among migrants with families apprehended by the US border patrol in the first eight months of 2018, Guatemalans had the largest share of any country).

Some researchers believe that Japan's collectivism may have its roots in the way rice is grown. Long-term collaboration is key when you want to succeed with rice: neighbours need to flood and drain their fields more or less in unison, and expensive irrigation systems are required, something that most individual villagers can't afford. You have to help each other and live in harmony.

Today, the Japanese proudly talk about their social capital, of which one manifestation is the existence of neighbourhood associations, which the locals call *chonaikai* or *jichikai*. The idea is that residents of a neighbourhood work together to make their community a better place, placemaking it—they organize festivals and sporting events, take care of clean-ups, patrol streets against crime, organize excursions for the elderly, hold regular lunch parties, and even exercise together doing *rajio taisō*—an exercise routine broadcasted early in the morning on the radio.

Across Japan there are about 300,000 neighbourhood associations—93 percent of locals claim their community has one, and if a neighbourhood association does exist, 94 percent of residents will belong to it. They talk about *chien*, or having a shared territorial bond, and believe in a "five-house rule" stating that you should keep a close relationship with people in the three houses opposite yours, as well as those who live in the house to your left and the one to your right. That's why it's not uncommon to spot a Japanese person cleaning up the sidewalk in front of other people's properties. Such commitment to community is also what's behind the next stop on my itinerary: a senior's club in Matsudo City.

Smile Muscles and Middle Class Mentality

The flat suburb of Tokyo, Matsudo, may be easy on the seniors' knees, but, I hear, gets pretty hot in the summer from all that asphalt everywhere. Matsudo is not Kyoto-pretty, yet it's ultra-clean and well organized. Plastic bags full of bottle caps hang in front of properties ready for recycling, pots of flowers are free of weeds and the sidewalks are nicely swept (signs of conscientiousness?).

As I approached a small parking lot, I saw a yellow board pinned to the railing. Glued to it were a few printouts advertising activities at a local senior's club. Monday: tarot reading and miso cooking. Tuesday: tai chi and flower pressing. Wednesday: more tai chi. Thursday: knitting. Friday: gardening. The club itself is located in a private house that has been adjusted to the needs of the elderly: there are all the requisite ramps as well as a stairlift chair. At the doors, I was greeted by Saitou-san, a cheerful middle-aged woman sporting jeans and a polyester apron, who owns the house and runs the club. I took off my shoes and replaced them with slippers that had been conveniently prepared for the guests, as is the Japanese custom, and followed Saitou-san to the second floor. The room up there smelled of roast pork and vegetables. Eighty-four-year-old Michiko was eating lunch with her friends, all of them elderly. That's what she came here for, she told me: friendship. "To move those muscles," she said, pointing to the part of her face that makes her lips lift in a smile. She made me think of that optimistic nun looking forward with "eager joy" to her vows at the School Sisters of Notre Dame.

After the women finished eating, which they did in relative silence (as is customary in Japan), they cleaned the table and set out to make pressed flower crafts, covering the tablecloth with perfectly dried petals. The conversation picked up, laced with laughter. Michiko told me that she liked making things with her own hands. "It keeps the brain stimulated," she said. Whether it was the friendships or the hobbies, she sure looked full of life and energy, despite her age.

Surveys show that just like Michiko, over 60 percent of Japanese seniors participate in some kind of social group activities, with hobby clubs being the most popular. Although these numbers are tricky to compare, in the US, for example, less than 20 percent of older adults attend seniors' centres on a regular basis. That's bad news. According to one study, going to such a centre even once a week lowers the risk of developing dementia by 40 percent. If each and every older adult in Canada picked up one social activity—be it pressing flowers, tai chi, or community gardening—the overall rate of Alzheimer's disease–related disabilities in the nation would decrease by over 16 percent.

What's more, senior Japanese have another advantage over their North American or British counterparts when it comes to longevity-boosting relationships—more of them stay married late into their lives. In Japan, almost 90 percent of men over the age of sixty-five have a wife, versus 73 percent in the UK, 68 percent in Canada, and roughly 70 percent in the US. For women, the rates are 56 percent (Japan) and 45 to 46 percent (UK, US, and Canada alike). There is a bit of a chicken-and-egg thing going on here, of course. Are more Japanese seniors married because their spouses live longer or do they live longer because they are married? The answer is—probably both.

One thing that kept coming up in my interviews with Japanese researchers, something that usually wasn't on the table when I talked with their Western colleagues, was the connection between longevity and egalitarianism. This topic often popped up right after the conversation covered the country's economic wealth and the social participation of seniors. "In Japan everybody has middle class mentality," regardless of their actual socio-economic class, says Shiro Horiuchi, a Tokyo-born longevity researcher who now works at the City University of New York. During the post-war economic growth in Japan, the income gap between the country's richest and poorest citizens flattened considerably—so much so that by the 1990s, over 90 percent of the people here considered themselves to be middle class.

Access to education and health care got levelled up, with obvious benefits to the well-being of the less wealthy. But it's not just that. The cultural differences and barriers between social classes, so prevalent in the US, are a rare thing in Japan, Horiuchi explained. There is a certain equality in Japan, with people easily interacting together— poor with the rich, underprivileged with powerful. That this boosts longevity and health of people with low socio-economic status is hardly surprising. When you feel your position in the society is strong, that you are important, that you belong, you experience less health-damaging uncertainty and stress. You may be a meagre gardener clipping public greenery, but you feel your role is vital for the greater good—and your greater psychological well-being translates into better physical fitness. One meta-analysis of studies conducted in eleven countries including Japan, Canada, and the US showed that each 0.05 unit increase in the Gini coefficient, a measure of income inequality, means 8 percent higher mortality risk. If the US (Gini index of 0.39) became as egalitarian as Iceland (0.24), Americans could basically give up on eating vegetables and still their longevity might not be any different than it is today.

What may be less apparent when it comes to the links between longevity and income equality is that living in an egalitarian society benefits the centenarian potential of the rich, too. In egalitarian countries, people trust each other and cooperate more. Those with money don't have to shut themselves off from the rest in gilded cages. There is no need to live in gated communities (which are a rare sight in Japan), to avoid walking the streets for security reasons, or to shun public transportation. This results in feelings of inclusion, harmony, and lowered anxiety for all. When there is social stratification, social capital erodes. People don't help each other much. They don't care about common goods the way the inhabitants of the longevity village, Matsukawa, care about their park with its foot-massage paths and flowers in the public toilets. They also don't feel inclined to work for the benefit of society long after they hit retirement age.

Working Till You Drop

I saw them everywhere across Japan, directing traffic around road construction sites, collecting parking fees, sweeping sidewalks in front of museums, and pruning roses in public parks: silver-hair employees doing their silver-hair jobs. According to governmental statistics, even among the seventy to seventy-four age group, one-third of men still work (and as many as 8 percent of those over eighty-five). They don't truly retire—they simply change careers to something easier, more relaxing. To find new jobs, they show up at places like the Silver Human Resources Center in Matsudo, one of over 1,300 senior employment agencies across the nation.

The centre is housed in a nondescript government building—it could be as well a place to get a driver's license or register a small business: glass doors that swoosh open to let you in, industrial carpeting on the floor silencing your steps, a few potted plants here and there. My attention was drawn to several boards that held pictures of elderly people on the job. There was a woman with a vacuum cleaner in what looked like a school classroom. A man fixing a bicycle. Someone—hard to tell the gender with all the protective gear—pruning a large tree. I was soon met by the director of the centre, an older man who himself might be already past retirement age. He told me they often have retired office workers come in, looking for something to fill up their days. Most people don't mind going from being high up the corporate ladder to sweeping streets, he told me. They just want something non-demanding that would make them feel useful. It's about social participation, he said, not money.

The oldest employee the Matsudo centre had recently matched with a job was already ninety-two—she works as a cleaner. But there are many, many others, some not much younger than her—parking attendants, gardeners, school-crossing patrollers. Work is something that gives structure to their life and roots them in the local community. Retiring, they feel, is losing something: their place in the society, meaning in life, respect. As many as 43 percent of Japanese workers say that retirement is something negative, compared to just 18 percent in the US and Canada. One famed Japanese longevity researcher, Shigeaki Hinohara, used to repeat: don't ever retire, but if you must, do so a lot later than age sixty-five. He stayed true to his words, working as long as eighteen hours a day until the day he passed away at the ripe age of 105.

Studies confirm the health benefits of staying busy well after the official retirement age. In one longitudinal survey, those seventy-five-year-olds who worked a paid job over a hundred hours a year in 1998 were more likely to be still alive in 2000, and in better health, than those who quit completely. Working past retirement may also be the reason why people in Nagano live so long—the prefecture boasts the highest employment rate of the elderly in the country. But if you are like me and don't find the idea of toiling well into your centenarian years all that appealing, rest assured: there is another lesson in here than just simply "work till you drop." Silver-hair jobs are good for health for several reasons: they encourage physical activity, lifelong learning, and making new friends. Above all, though, they are about ikigai.

Ikigai is a word you hear a lot in Japan. I hear it when I talk to Michiko as she presses flowers at the senior's club, from Fujita Masatoshi, the non-retired gardener, and from many other seniors and non-seniors alike. Ikigai does not have a perfect equivalent in English, but is often translated either as "purpose in life" or "life worth living." Among Japanese people over the age of sixty-five, about 88 percent claim to have ikigai.

If you are a Westerner, you may be tempted to see ikigai as self-fulfillment, but that's not exactly it. It's more about how you help others, contribute to the society—which was evident to me from the way the Japanese people I met talked about ikigai. Yet since the word doesn't translate easily, there are no studies that directly compare Japan with other nations on ikigai. One study that came close asked people in ten countries to rate such statements as "I am doing something useful for my family or for the world" or "My family or others believe I am able to do something important for them." Japan scored the highest in terms of the percentage of people who answered "very much" to these claims—27 and 26 percent, respectively. In the US, those numbers were 11 percent for the first question and a mere 8 percent for the second.

Those I talked to in Japan told me that for them ikigai is "making others happy," "helping others," "making people laugh," and "raising children." No matter what your particular ikigai is, though, research suggests that it improves physical well-being and extends life. In a study that followed over forty thousand Japanese for seven years, among people who had ikigai at day one, only 12 percent rated their health as "poor" later on, compared to 46 percent of those who didn't have purpose in life. What's more, those with ikigai were 50 percent less likely to die compared to the rest—an effect similar to quitting smoking and far stronger than that of becoming a gym bunny. No wonder, then, that the Japanese Ministry of Health,

Labour, and Welfare has included ikigai in their health promotion strategy.

Although ikigai is a particularly important part of the Japanese culture that contributes to longevity, other traditions and concepts likely boost the health of the locals, too. I'm talking about things like *chado*, haiku, *shodo, ikebana,* and *hanami.*

Jumping Frogs and Forgotten Umbrellas

Clad in a silvery-pink kimono that reminds me of cherry blossoms, Chiaki-san, my hostess at a Kyoto teahouse, wiped porcelain bowls with a delicate silk cloth, then reached for a bamboo ladle to pour hot water into them. All her movements were precise, deliberate yet artful, her hands dancing over the dishes. I was trying to concentrate on the simple beauty of the tea ceremony, to clear my mind, but I wasn't used to sitting on my legs on tatami mats. Soon, I started to fidget.

The chado, or tea ceremony, I was participating in was a shortened, one-hour version of a ritual that normally lasts four times as long. It's supposed to promote inner peace, so talking is discouraged. Every detail counts: the direction in which the bowls face, the placement of the tatami mats, and the position of the calligraphy scroll hanging on the wall. As I watched Chiaki-san mix the powdered green matcha tea with water, the silence broken only by the quick swish-swish-swish of her bamboo whisk, I began to relax, my breathing slowing down. I have to admit: observing the studied movements of the hostess was mesmerizing.

Tea ceremony, just like the Japanese art of flower arrangement (ikebana) or cherry tree viewing (hanami), is all about mindfulness: attention to the present, clearing the mind. Japanese culture abounds in traditions that centre on the appreciation of nature and beauty, promoting moment-to-moment awareness. There is shodo,

Japanese calligraphy, which treasures harmony, simplicity, and aesthetic pleasures. There is *bonsai*, growing dwarf trees in earthenware pots, a time-consuming, patience-requiring art. Hanami, or cherry tree viewing, is also, in a way, about mindfulness, since the stunning glory of the pink blooms is very fleeting, lasting only a couple of days. And then there is haiku, poetry that is so simple that it can feel like meditation. The idea is to capture a moment in a mere seventeen syllables. Here is probably the most famous haiku, a seventeenth-century verse called the frog haiku:

> *An old pond*
> *a frog jumps*
> *the sound of water*

It's so Zen, I can almost feel my telomeres extending from reading this. As you probably suspect, Zen is another keyword here. Zen, a school of Buddhism that originated in China, lies at the heart of Japanese culture, promoting self-control, meditation, and self-discovery. One old story I've read recently in a BBC article by Steve John Powell (and originally coming from Paul Reps' 1957 anthology of Zen texts, *Zen Flesh, Zen Bones*), is particularly good at explaining what Zen is about:

> After studying to be a Zen teacher for many years, Teno went to visit Nan-in, an old Zen master. It was raining heavily and, as is customary, Teno left his clogs and umbrella in the entrance before entering Nan-in's house. After greeting each other, Nan-in asked Teno: "Did you leave your umbrella to the left or right of your clogs?" Unable to answer, Teno realized he was still a long way from attaining Zen, and went away to study for six more years.

If you are anything like me and sometimes have no idea how you got home from work, even though you obviously did drive and did not crash the car, perfect Zen is far more than six years away. Yet it's still worth pursuing it—Zen meditation experts have longer telomeres than those who don't follow the practice. Zen meditation also increases heart rate variability and helps with pain. Just like mindfulness meditation, Zen and its cousin traditions such as chado tea ceremony, ikebana flower arranging, or haiku poetry act against stress and anxiety, calming the mind and hence, in all likelihood, promoting physical health (although, admittedly, no one seems to have studied the telomere length of ikebana or haiku practitioners).

Yet just as Japanese traditions of tea drinking are changing—Chiaki-san tells me most people simply use teabags on an everyday basis and do chado only once a year or so—so does the society itself, with potential longevity consequences. First, there are the physical issues. Remember Okinawa and how everyone used to obsess about the health-boosting lifestyle of its inhabitants? Well, it's all over now: these inhabitants are no longer the longevity champions of Japan. They've developed a penchant for Western-style fast foods and their well-being has nosedived. But there are other threats to Japanese longevity besides burgers. Social inequalities are increasing and people are overworked and under-slept, so much so that they have no time for romantic relationships—or even for sex. Among those who are not married, roughly 40 percent are still virgins at the age of thirty-four. In one admittedly smallish poll—it involved six hundred men in their forties—well over a half reported having "zero sex." Just like sex, marriage is often not happening, either. Loneliness is rampant. In every other developed country, the number of teenagers who claim to be lonely hovers somewhere in the single digits. In Japan, it's 30 percent. That's not good for anyone's telomeres.

Meanwhile, some researchers claim that the famed Japanese collectivism may be also on the decline, as the young, influenced by the West, get more and more individualistic. The Gini index has been climbing steadily as income inequalities deepen, too. No one knows, of course, how exactly these changes may impact Japanese longevity.

In twenty or fifty years, will Japan still be the longest-living nation on the planet? It's important to remember that the people who are now reaching their hundredth birthdays have lived in a Japan that was more collectivistic, more egalitarian, and less fast-paced than it is today. Will their great-grandchildren have similar chances of becoming centenarians?

Despite these potential anti-longevity trends, there are still many health-related lessons we can learn from the Japanese. We can eat less meat—or none at all—more vegetables, and more soy, and we can walk often and do yearly dry dock checkups. Most importantly, though, we can take to heart the Japanese saying, "sickness and health start with the mind."

It might be tempting to look at the Japanese mindset and try to replicate it at home. But culture is not a book we can just borrow. Some things simply won't work if transplanted wholesale from one country to another. We can try all we might, but the UK, Canada, or the US won't suddenly become collectivist cultures. Yet what we can do is change our focus a bit from inward to outward, from an "I" mentality to a "we" one. We could think a little less about our own individual achievements and status and more about social harmony and finding a place for ourselves in the community. We could try to temper the "me, me, me culture" and concentrate more on the group.

You don't need to move to Nagano to extend your life, and without revising your values and attitudes, it might have not worked anyway. But you can commit yourself to making your current home a bit more like the longevity village, Matsukawa, with its gleaming public spaces designed to include everyone, where even kindergarteners are safe to walk on their own. Why not set up an informal neighbourhood association, for example? Have regular meetings to discuss the needs of the community and to organize clean-ups, block parties, and sporting events. Exercising together at the break of dawn to the radio may feel quite weird, but a jogging group might work, or driveway basketball meet-ups. Following the Japanese five-house rule is a good idea, too—so if you don't know the names of your neighbours in three houses in front of yours and in those to the sides, go out and introduce yourself.

Learning longevity lessons from the cherry blossom land does not mean you need to work till you drop at 105, either. What it does mean is that finding something larger than yourself to fill your days once you retire is a good idea. Don't just mope around the house with the TV as your companion—volunteer, get a hobby (and one that benefits others would be best), and involve yourself more with your family and friends. That said, discovering your ikigai, your purpose in life, is probably the top advice you should take from the Japanese—and it may be easier to do so if you calm your mind first with Zen-related practices. That's something you can transplant from Japan directly—meditate, try ikebana, or write a haiku. And if a tea ceremony does not sound appealing, develop your own food-related traditions—a coffee ceremony, perhaps?—making sure they are slow and mindful. Even replacing your coffee-to-go with a European-style pause at a café could make a difference: after all, the idea here it to be present in the moment, noting the feel of the cup, the taste and smell of the liquid, the sounds around you.

One health-boosting and life-extending lesson that will certainly not be easy to follow is making our societies more egalitarian. Unless you are the current president of the United States or someone with similar power, you can't, of course, transform your country with a few simple decisions. You can, however, try to open yourself up to those outside of your social class. Talk to them and respect them. Think how your decisions may affect their lives. Donate money and time. And, of course, there is also your vote. Use it wisely—it can impact your centenarian potential and that of your children.

As for policy makers, Shiro Horiuchi believes that they should strive to make disadvantaged people belong in the society. "I feel that in the US the thinking behind health care policy is relatively mechanical: more money, more materials, people will be happy. But more thought should be given to making underprivileged people feel more integrated in the society," he says. In other words: it's not enough to throw cash around on drugs or new scanners. If you want to extend longevity in a country, you need to trim the cultural barriers between the poor and the rich, and help the former develop stronger feelings of belonging. Admittedly, buying medical equipment is far easier than pushing for social equality—just as taking wonder-diet supplements is easier than improving relationships. Yet if longevity is truly the goal, it's all worth it.

A FEW SUGGESTIONS TO BOOST YOUR LONGEVITY

Focus outward rather than inward—try to think about the needs of other people around you more often. Participate in your neighbourhood associations. Follow the five-house rule—keep a close relationship with people in the three houses opposite yours and those who live in the house to your left and the one to your right. Find your ikigai—purpose in life. Value your work, and if you are retired, make sure to find yourself something to keep you busy and useful to society. Try to find zen—meditate or do haiku or ikebana. Like the Japanese, enjoy simple things.

EPILOGUE

WHAT TO DO TO LIVE LONG? From fountain-searching Ponce de Léon to pill-popping techies from Silicon Valley, humanity has been trying to pinpoint the answer for centuries, often fixating on all the wrong things: miracle diets, miracle foods, miracle supplements. We skip gluten and invest in exercise gadgets. We swallow vitamins. We obsess about BMI. Yet even though healthy nutrition and physical activity are indeed important for health—within reason—there are things that can affect your centenarian potential even more, things that we all too often sacrifice while we chase fad diets and the newest cardio workouts. Friendships. Purpose in life. Empathy. Kindness. Science shows that these "soft" health drivers are often more powerful than diet and exercise. Admittedly, without the right genetic makeup you are unlikely to beat the longevity record of Jeanne Calment, no matter how much you volunteer or how great your marriage is, but if you focus on your relationships and your mind, you may still considerably slow down your epigenetic clock and add many years to your life.

We humans are social apes. Over the course of evolution, we've developed several intertwined systems that regulate our social lives on one hand and our physiology on the other. The amygdala, the insula, the social hormones, the vagus nerve, the HPA axis—all of these link our bodies and our minds, contributing to our centenarian potential. We feel safe when we are surrounded by friendly others. The nervous system, the gastrointestinal system, the immune system—all of these function properly when the tribe is there for us and when we are there for the tribe. Involved in a group, we flourish.

What's more, focusing your longevity effort on growing as a person could not just add years to your life but also make that life more worth living. Caring for others, contributing to the community, and living meaningfully help us reach old age, stave off disease, and make us happy all at the same time. One could argue, of course, that volunteering or community-making in order to get healthier is egoistic and untoward. I don't agree with that view. Even if that first impulse to lead a kinder life is indeed egoistic, I believe that for most people, taking a deeper look at how they spend their time and participate in their society can help them change for the better. And as a result, we could all end up living in a place that's worth living in.

Think about it—do you want to spend a hundred years in a society where everyone cares about nothing but themselves? Do you want to live on a planet that's in the throes of climate change, bashed with extreme weather and conflicts over resources? Boosting empathy can both make us healthier and make our planet healthier, too—studies show, for example, that high empathy motivates people to fight climate change. Conscientiousness also often means environmental engagement. If we invest more in being kind, mindful, and conscientious we are more likely to improve the conditions in which we all live. Besides, if we ruin the earth, we may never make it as centenarians anyway. Hurricanes and wildfires don't care about your diet. Wars kill people with low cholesterol, too.

For all the above reasons, it's vital that we recognize the role the human psyche plays in longevity. Policymakers are beginning to focus their attention on issues such as loneliness and divorce rates—yet they still mostly see them as social problems, not public health issues. That should change. Loneliness is a mortality risk as much as poor nutrition, if not more so. We should identify populations of concern and aim our efforts at prevention. We could, for instance, help isolated seniors find their way back into society by encouraging volunteering or setting up hobby clubs. We could offer paid maternity and paternity leaves to support early family bonding. We could draft guidelines recommending regular social activity ("at least 150 minutes of fun with friends every week"?). And maybe our schools should teach children empathy as much as they should teach them about nutrition.

We invest so much money in expensive clinical trials that promise extravagant therapies to reverse aging. We put our hopes in young blood transfusions and rejuvenating mitochondria. But maybe we should just do things that are already known to work, such as volunteering, making friends, and learning optimism. Over the years I have been guilty of many dietary and fitness obsessions myself, but I'm trying to change. I have stopped worrying that most of what I eat is not organic, and I don't scour the internet for new recipes that would hike our family's turmeric intake. Instead of running several miles a fourth time in a week, I may now plop down on the couch beside my husband and pull out a card game. I invest more time into my marriage. I stop to chat with neighbours. I try to be kinder. In all fairness, I have no idea whether my telomeres are shrinking more slowly, but let me tell you: no amount of spinach has ever made me feel this good.

It's time we recognize that improving our social lives and cultivating our minds can be at least as important for health and longevity as are diet and exercise. When you grow as a person, chances are, you will also grow young. To Michael Pollan's famous statement, "Eat food. Not too much. Mostly plants," I would add: "Be social, care for others, enjoy life."

INTRODUCTION

2   *A recent review of almost a hundred studies showed that people who have a BMI (body mass index) of 30 to 35 . . .* —A word on mortality risk. Throughout this book, you will see me referring to "lower mortality risk." What that essentially means (without going too much into mathematical subtleties) is that within the follow-up period of a particular study—say, 5 years or 10 years or 25—particular people were less likely to die. If, for example, mortality risk in some study was 20 percent lower for people who did X, this means that people who did X were estimated to be approximately 20 percent less likely to die than they normally would in the period in which the scientists followed up on them.

3   *Studies show that building a strong support network of family and friends lowers mortality risk by about 45 percent.* —Julianne Holt-Lunstad, David A. Sbarra and Theodore F. Robles, "Advancing Social Connection as a Public Health Priority in the United States," *American Psychologist* 72 (2017).

3   *Exercise, on the other hand, can lower mortality risk by 23 to 33 percent.* —Ralph S. Paffenbarger et al., "The Association of Changes in Physical-Activity Level and Other Lifestyle Characteristics with Mortality among Men," 328 (1993): 538-545 AND Marc Nocon et al., "Association of physical activity with all-cause and cardiovascular mortality: a systematic review and meta-analysis," *European Journal of Preventive Cardiology* 15 (2008).

3   *Eating six or more servings of vegetables and fruits per day, which is admittedly quite a lot, can cut mortality risk by 26 percent.* —Xia Wang et al., "Fruit and vegetable consumption and mortality from all causes, cardiovascular disease, and cancer: systematic review and dose-response meta-analysis of prospective cohort studies," *BMJ* 349 (2014).

3   *. . . following the Mediterranean diet—eating lots of fruits, vegetables, and whole grains, replacing butter with olive oil, etc.—21 percent.* —Panagiota N. Mitrou et al., "Mediterranean Dietary Pattern and Prediction of All-Cause Mortality in a US Population," *JAMA Internal Medicine* 167 (2007): 2461-2468.

4   *Among the French, 61 percent of those in their thirties and forties eat dinner with their family, at the table, each and every day.* —"Les Repas Traditionnel Fait de la

Resistance!" BVA, accessed November 29, 2017, http://www.bva.fr/fr/sondages/le_repas_traditionnel_fait_de_la_resistance.html

4 *Now compare that to the mere 24 percent of Americans that age who do so . . .* —"Are Americans Still Serving Up Family Dinners?," The Harris Poll, accessed November 29, 2017, http://www.theharrispoll.com/health-and-life/Are_Americans_Still_Serving_Up_Family_Dinners_.html

6 *A committed romantic relationship, which according to some studies can lower your mortality risk by a staggering 49 percent.* —Julianne Holt-Lunstad, David A. Sbarra and Theodore F. Robles, "Advancing Social Connection as a Public Health Priority in the United States," *American Psychologist* 72 (2017).

6 *. . . having a conscientious personality (44 percent).* —Eileen K. Graham et al., "Personality Predicts Mortality Risk: An Integrative Data Analysis of 15 International Longitudinal Studies," *Journal of Research in Personality* (2017).

6 *. . . volunteering—about 22 to 44 percent . . .* —Doug Oman, Carl Thoresen and Kay Mcmahon, "Volunteerism and Mortality among the Community-dwelling Elderly," *Journal of Health Psychology* 4 (1999).

6 *. . . omega-3s—no effects found.* Lee Hooper et al., "Risks and benefits of omega 3 fats for mortality, cardiovascular disease, and cancer: systematic review," *BMJ* 332 (2006).

7 *In one particularly striking study, researchers evaluated aging biomarkers in almost a thousand New Zealanders . . .* —Daniel W. Belsky et al., "Eleven Telomere, Epigenetic Clock, and Biomarker-Composite Quantifications of Biological Aging: Do They Measure the Same Thing?," *American Journal of Epidemiology* 187 (2018): 1220-1230.

8 *Former president Barack Obama noted that "we live in a culture that discourages empathy."* —"Obama to Graduates: Cultivate Empathy," Northwestern University, accessed August 1, 2019, https://www.northwestern.edu/newscenter/stories/2006/06/barack.html

8 *In 2018 then British prime minister Theresa May appointed a "minister for loneliness" to deal with what she dubbed "the sad reality of modern life" . . .* —Peter Walker, "May appoints minister to tackle loneliness issues raised by Jo Cox," *The Guardian*, accessed August 12, 2019, https://www.theguardian.com/society/2018/jan/16/may-appoints-minister-tackle-loneliness-issues-raised-jo-cox

8 *He admitted, though, that "many clinicians aren't clear about the strong connection between loneliness and the very health problems we are trying to address, often with medications and procedures."* —Jena McGregor, "This former surgeon general says there's a 'loneliness epidemic' and work is partly to blame," *The Washington Post*, accessed August 12, 2019, https://www.washingtonpost.com/news/on-leadership/wp/2017/10/04/this-former-surgeon-general-says-theres-a-loneliness-epidemic-and-work-is-partly-to-blame/

PART I: THE MIND-BODY CONNECTION AND ITS LONGEVITY CONSEQUENCES

CHAPTER 1: IS DEATH OPTIONAL?

14 *Unfortunately, as one researcher aptly put it, "In our experience, claims to age 130 exist only where records do not."* —Robert D. Young et al., "Typologies of Extreme Longevity Myths," *Current Gerontology and Geriatrics Research* 2010 (2010).

14 *When in 2016 several scientists published a paper claiming that the maximum human lifespan fluctuates around 115 . . .* —Xiao Dong, Brandon Milholland and Jan Vijg, "Evidence for a limit to human lifespan," *Nature* 538 (2016): 257-259.

16 *. . . which, in case you are wondering, has been verified and established beyond doubt.* —Jean-Marie Robine and Michel Allard, "The oldest human," *Science* 279 (1998): 1834–1835.

16 *Even the* New York Times *fell for it, reporting in her obituary that she "only quit smoking five years ago."* —Craig R. Whitney, "Jeanne Calment, World's Elder, Dies at 122," *The New York Times*, August 5, 1997.

17 *While a regular Joe or Sue will spend almost 18 percent of their time on earth overtaken by disease . . .* —Stacy L. Andersen et al., "Health Span Approximates Life Span Among Many Supercentenarians: Compression of Morbidity at the Approximate Limit of Life Span," *The Journals of Gerontology* Series A, 67A (2012): 395-405.

18 *For most of us, how long we live is only about 20 to 25 percent heritable.* —Anatoliy I. Yashin et al., "Joint influence of small-effect genetic variants on human longevity," *Aging* 2 (2010): 612-620.

19 *One study showed that if kept in petri dishes, away from predators and other environmental dangers . . .* —Ralf Schaible et al., "Constant mortality and fertility over age in *Hydra*," *PNAS* 112 (2015): 15701-15706.

23 *Thanks to recent studies, however, we now know that the biggest difference in telomere length . . .* —Sonja Entringer et al., "The fetal programming of telomere biology hypothesis: an update," *Philosophical Transactions* B 373 (2018).

28 *. . . which came up in data from many historical famines, including the Ukrainian famine of 1933 and the Irish one of 1845 to 1849.* —Virginia Zarulli et al., "Women live longer than men even during severe famines and epidemics," *PNAS* 115 (2018): E832-E840.

28 *Researchers have calculated that among the Donner party, the male mortality risk was almost double the female one.* —Donald K. Grayson, "Human Mortality in a Natural Disaster: The Willie Handcart Company," *Journal of Anthropological Research* 52 (1996): 185-205.

28 *When German researchers looked at over eleven thousand Catholic nuns and monks from Bavarian cloisters . . .* —Marc Luy, "Causes of Male Excess Mortality: Insights from Cloistered Populations," *Population and Development Review* 29 (2003): 647-676.

28 *In a comparison of fifty-nine species inhabiting zoos, only four had males that outlived the females.* —Morgane Tidière et al., "Comparative analyses of longevity and

senescence reveal variable survival benefits of living in zoos across mammals," *Scientific Reports* 6 (2016).

29   *An analysis of lifespans of eunuchs living in nineteenth-century Korean courts . . .* —Kyung-Jin Min, Cheol-Koo Lee and Han-Nam Park, "The lifespan of Korean eunuchs," *Current Biology* 22 (2012): R792-R793.

29   *What eunuchs are short on, of course, is testosterone . . .* —Rita Ostan et al., "Gender, aging and longevity in humans: an update of an intriguing/neglected scenario paving the way to a gender-specific medicine," *Clinical Science* 130 (2016): 1711-1725.

29   *On the other hand, female hormones such as estrogens give a boost to the immune system . . .* —ibid.

29   *In an interview for The New Yorker back in 2017 . . .* —Tad Friend, "Silicon Valley's Quest to Live Forever," *The New Yorker*, accessed July 25, 2019, https://www.newyorker.com/magazine/2017/04/03/silicon-valleys-quest-to-live-forever

30   *There is growing evidence that metformin may indeed prolong life and delay aging . . .* —Nir Barzilai et al., "Metformin as a Tool to Target Aging," *Cell Metabolism* 23 (2016): 1060-1065.

30   *In an interview for* Scientific American, *one University of California molecular biologist said it "just reeks of snake oil."* —Rebecca Robbins, "Young-Blood Transfusions Are on the Menu at Society Gala," *Scientific American*, accessed July 25, 2019, https://www.scientificamerican.com/article/young-blood-transfusions-are-on-the-menu-at-society-gala/

CHAPTER 2: HOW YOUR MIND TALKS WITH YOUR BODY

34   *In experiments, people who merely imagine exercising their hand muscles end up with improved strength.* —Brian C. Clark et al., "The power of the mind: the cortex as a critical determinant of muscle strength/weakness," *Journal of Neurophysiology* 112 (2014): 3219-3226.

34   *Others get real rashes from exposure to fake poison ivy.* —Sandra Blakeslee, "Placebos Prove So Powerful Even Experts Are Surprised; New Studies Explore the Brain's Triumph Over Reality," *The New York Times*, accessed July 25, 2019, https://www.nytimes.com/1998/10/13/science/placebos-prove-so-powerful-even-experts-are-surprised-new-studies-explore-brain.html

34   *Placebo treatments, meanwhile, are so effective that 42 percent of balding men maintain or increase hair growth after such "cures."* —ibid.

34   *Hypnosis can even be used to reduce pain during lumbar punctures . . ."* —Christina Liossi and Popi Hatira, "Clinical hypnosis in the alleviation of procedure-related pain in pediatric oncology patients," *International Journal of Clinical and Experimental Hypnosis* 51 (2003): 4-28.

34   *. . . and heart surgeries.* —Edwin J. Weinstein and Phillip K. Au, "Use of hypnosis before and during angioplasty," *American Journal of Clinical Hypnosis* 34 (1991): 29-37.

34 *William Paul Young, a Canadian novelist, once wrote that "emotions are the colors of the soul"* . . . —Young, William Paul. *The Shack* (London: Hodder & Stoughton, 2007).

36 *It was about ten o'clock at night when SM* . . . —Justin S. Feinstein et al., "The Human Amygdala and the Induction and Experience of Fear," *Current Biology* 21 (2011): 34-38.

39 *During World War Two, rumours abounded that the Nazis were developing a miracle cure for stress* . . . —Christoper M. Burns, "The History of Cortisone Discovery and Development," in *Corticosteroids: An Issue of Rheumatic Disease Clinics of North America*, ed. Marcy B. Bolster (Philadelphia: Elsevier, 2016), 1-15.

40 *When the scientists visited her room in Saint Mary's Hospital in Rochester, Minnesota, they found her exercising* . . . —Rooke, Thom. *The Quest for Cortisone* (East Lansing, Michigan: Michigan State University Press, 2012).

42 *The hypothalamus begins to shrink* . . . —Teresa E. Seeman et al., "Price of Adaptation—Allostatic Load and Its Health Consequences," *JAMA Internal Medicine* 157 (1997): 2259-2268.

42 *Since cortisol takes up fat from places such as the legs and arms* . . . —A. Steptoe and J. Wardle, "Cardiovascular stress responsivity, body mass and abdominal adiposity," *International Journal of Obesity* 29 (2005): 1329-1337.

42 *Like a finger on a light switch, stress hormones turn genes on and off.* —David Muehsam et al., "The embodied mind: A review on functional genomic and neurological correlates of mind-body therapies," *Neuroscience and Biobehavioral Reviews* 73 (2017): 165-181.

43 *This so-called "sickness behavior" is actually caused by your own immune system, or your pro-inflammatory cytokines, to be precise.* —Robert Dantzer, "Cytokine, Sickness Behavior, and Depression," *Neurologic Clinics* 24 (2006): 441-460.

44 *One meta-analysis showed that about a quarter of patients with hepatitis C* . . . —Marc Udina et al., "Interferon- induced depression in chronic hepatitis C: a systematic review and meta-analysis," *The Journal of Clinical Psychiatry* 73 (2012): 1128–1138.

44 *In animals, injections with both infectious bacteria and pro-inflammatory cytokines cause depression, too.* —Julie E. Finnell and Susan K. Wood, "Neuroinflammation at the interface of depression and cardiovascular disease: Evidence from rodent models of social stress," *Neurobiology of Stress* 4 (2016): 1-14.

44 *Studies on mice and rats show that only those who are susceptible to stress and deal with challenges passively* . . . —ibid.

44 *For this reason anti-inflammatory drugs are now being proposed as treatment for depression in patients who don't respond to traditional treatments.* —Ole Köhler et al., "Inflammation in Depression and the Potential for Anti-Inflammatory Treatment," *Current Neuropharmacology* 14 (2016): 732-742.

45 *About 10 to 15 percent of people who die plunging into an ocean or a river have no water in their lungs* . . . —Philippe Lunetta, Jerome Modelland Antti Sajantila, "What Is the Incidence and Significance of "Dry-Lungs" in Bodies Found in Water?" *The American Journal of Forensic Medicine and Pathology* 25 (2004): 291-301.

45 *In animal experiments similar cases have been attributed to the overstimulation of the vagus nerve.* —Paolo Alboni, Marco Alboni and Lorella Gianfranchi, "Simultaneous occurrence of two independent vagal reflexes: a possible cause of vagal sudden death," *Heart* 97 (2011): 623-625.

45 *Such sudden vagal death, some scientists believe, could also explain the mortal power of voodoo curses.* —ibid.

46 *Some research actually suggests that we could even treat chronic pain and depression by applying electrical stimulation to the vagus nerve.* —A.J. Rush et al., "Vagus nerve stimulation (VNS) for treatment-resistant depressions: a multicenter study," *Biological Psychiatry* 47 (2000): 276–286.

47 *. . . and even an earlier death.* —Julian Thayer et al., "A meta-analysis of heart rate variability and neuroimaging studies: Implications for heart rate variability as a marker of stress and health," *Neuroscience and Biobehavioral Reviews* 36 (2012): 747-756.

47 *Luckily for me studies show that lifestyle changes, such as yoga, can improve HRV quickly . . .* —Marian Papp et al., "Increased heart rate variability but no effect on blood pressure from 8 weeks of hatha yoga—a pilot study," *BMC Research Notes* 6 (2013).

49 *One such study showed, for example, that roller derby players exchange microbes with opposing teams during tournaments.* —James Meadow et al., "Significant changes in the skin microbiome mediated by the sport of roller derby," *PeerJ* 1 (2013): e53.

49 *Family members, meanwhile, share bacteria with each other and even their dogs.* —Se Jin Song et al., "Cohabiting family members share microbiota with one another and with their dogs," *eLife* 2 (2013): e00458.

49 *If you breed mice devoid of any beneficial gut bacteria, the rodents will be loners, preferring to sit away from all the others.* —L. Desbonnet et al., "Microbiota is essential for social development in the mouse," *Molecular Psychiatry* 19 (2014): 146-148.

50 *And if you recolonize their intestines with microbes, their personality will change once again—back to social.* —ibid.

50 *Germ-free rodents have been shown to have overreactive HPA axes and to be less resilient to stress.* —Timothy G. Dinan et al., "Collective unconscious: How gut microbes shape human behavior," *Journal of Psychiatric Research* 63 (2015): 1-9.

50 *In the Philippines, for instance, young people in their twenties who had a lot of contact with animal feces . . .* —Thomas W. McDade et al., "Do environments in infancy moderate the association between stress and inflammation in adulthood? Initial evidence from a birth cohort in the Philippines," *Brain, Behavior, and Immunity* 31 (2013): 23-30.

50 *When a group of American volunteers drank probiotic-rich fermented milk for about a month . . .* —Kirsten Tillisch et al., "Consumption of Fermented Milk Product With Probiotic Modulates Brain Activity," *Gastroenterology* 144 (2013): 1394-1401.e4.

50 *A similar experiment showed that consumption of the bacteria* Bifidobacterium longum . . . —Michaël Messaoudi et al., "Beneficial psychological effects of a probiotic formulation (*Lactobacillus helveticus* R0052 and *Bifidobacterium longum* R0175) in healthy human volunteers," *Gut Microbes* 4 (2011): 256-261.

50   *In one particularly revealing study scientists have taken stool from depressed patients . . .*
     —John R. Kelly, "Transferring the blues: depression-associated gut microbiota
     induces neurobehavioural changes in the rat," *Journal of Psychiatric Research* 82
     (2016): 109–118.

50   *Take poop from an anxious mouse and insert it into a second mouse, and your mouse
     number two will become anxious as well.* —P. Bercik et al., "The intestinal micro-
     biota affect central levels of brain-derived neurotropic factor and behavior in
     mice," *Gastroenterology* 141 (2011): 599-609.

51   *When experimental animals are stressed, the composition of germs in their poop changes
     in response . . .* —Eoin Sherwin, Timothy G. Dinan and John F. Cryan, "Recent
     developments in understanding the role of the gut microbiota in brain health
     and disease," *Annals of the New York Academy of Sciences* 1420 (2018): 5-25.

52   *When researchers from the Max Planck Institute for Biology of Aging in Germany
     made middle-aged turquoise killifish nibble on the feces of their younger companions . . .*
     —Patrick Smith et al., "Regulation of life span by the gut microbiota in the
     short-lived African turquoise killifish," *eLife* 6 (2017): e27014.

52   *Mr. Wright had cancer.* —C.R. Snyder, Lori Irving and John Anderson, "Hope
     and Health," in *Handbook of Social and Clinical Psychology: The Health Perspective*,
     eds. C. R. Snyder and D. R. Forsyth (Elmsford, NY, US: Pergamon Press, 1991),
     285-305.

53   *In one study of cancer survivors suffering from fatigue . . .* —Teri W. Hoenemeyer et
     al., "Open-Label Placebo Treatment for Cancer-Related Fatigue: A Randomized-
     Controlled Clinical Trial," *Scientific Reports* 8 (2018).

54   *When scientists put people who have received placebos into functional magnetic resonance
     imaging scanners . . .* —L.Y. Atlas and T.D. Wager, "A Meta-analysis of Brain Mecha-
     nisms of Placebo Analgesia: Consistent Findings and Unanswered Questions,"
     in: *Placebo*, eds. Fabrizio Benedetti et al. (Berlin: Springer, 2014): 37–69.

CHAPTER 3: A SNIFF OF LOVE

57   *According to the producer's website, OxyLuv is supposed to "create feelings of trust
     between others" and reduce my "social fears, anxiety, stress."* —PherLuv Pheromone
     Molecule Compounds, accessed July 29, 2019, https://www.pherluv.com/
     index.php/oxytocin-nasal-spray

58   *They incite male cichlid fish to be better fathers.* —Lauren A.O'Connell· Bryan
     J.Matthews and Hans A.Hofmann, "Isotocin regulates paternal care in a monog-
     amous cichlid fish," *Hormones and Behavior* 61 (2012): 725-733.

58   *According to one theory called "the neurochemical hypothesis for the origin of homi-
     nids"* —Mary Ann Raghanti et al., "A neurochemical hypothesis for the origin
     of hominids," *PNAS* 115 (2018): E1108-E1116.

60   *. . . since late Pleistocene times, approximately thirty thousand years ago, they've actually
     slightly shrunk by about 10 percent.* —Jean-Jacques Hublin, Simon Neubauer and
     Philipp Gunz, "Brain ontogeny and life history in Pleistocene hominins," *Phil-
     osophical Transactions of The Royal Society* B 370 (2015).

60 *Scientists believe that what may be responsible for such side effects, be it smaller brains or white forehead patches, is the neural crest.* —Brian Hare, "Survival of the Friendliest: *Homo sapiens* Evolved via Selection for Prosociality," *The Annual Review of Psychology* 68 (2017): 155-186.

61 *And, in their brains they have twice as much serotonin, one of the social neuropeptides . . .* —Cheryl D. Stimpson et al., "Differential serotonergic innervation of the amygdala in bonobos and chimpanzees," *Social Cognitive and Affective Neuroscience* 11 (2016): 413-422.

61 *Yet in the case of our ancestors, Wrangham argues . . .* Wrangham, Richard. *The Goodness Paradox: The Strange Relationship Between Virtue and Violence in Human Evolution* (New York: Pantheon Books, 2019), 47-65.

62 *Over our evolutionary history, selecting for more friendly hominins . . .* —In the language of paleoanthropology the word "hominin" stands for modern humans and all extinct species closely related to us.

63 *And while prairie vole parents take care of their little ones together, with the fathers licking and grooming the kids . . .* —Manal Tabbaa et al., "Neuropeptide Regulation of Social Attachment: The Prairie Vole Model," *Comprehensive Physiology* 7 (2016): 81-104.

63 *. . . the monogamous voles have a very different pattern of oxytocin and vasopressin receptors in their brains as compared to their promiscuous cousins . . .* —Manal Tabbaa et al., "Neuropeptide Regulation of Social Attachment: The Prairie Vole Model," *Comprehensive Physiology* 7 (2016): 81-104.

65 *. . . as one 2017 study has found, is connected to the so-called pro-sociality gene, GTF2I . . .* —T.L. Procyshyn et al., "The Williams syndrome prosociality gene *GTF2I* mediates oxytocin reactivity and social anxiety in a healthy population," *Biology Letters* 13 (2017).

65 *Mice that don't have oxytocin receptor genes tend to behave in autistic ways . . .* —Mauricio Aspé-Sánchez et al., "Oxytocin and Vasopressin Receptor Gene Polymorphisms: Role in Social and Psychiatric Traits," *Frontiers in Neuroscience* 9 (2016).

65 *Also, some experiments have shown that spraying oxytocin into the noses of kids with autism may boost their social skills.* —Takamitsu Watanabe et al., "Clinical and neural effects of six-week administration of oxytocin on core symptoms of autism," *Brain* 11 (2015): 3400–3412.

65 *Research shows that people with an AA variant of an oxytocin receptor gene called* rs53576 *are less empathic . . .* —Franz Korbinian Huetter et al., "Association of a Common Oxytocin Receptor Gene Polymorphism with Self-Reported 'Empathic Concern' in a Large Population of Healthy Volunteers," *PLOS One* (2016).

65 *. . . as one study found, if they are mothers, parent their kids with less sensitivity in times of parental conflict.* —Melissa L. Sturge-Apple and Dante Cicchetti, "Differential Susceptibility in Spillover Between Interparental Conflict and Maternal Parenting Practices: Evidence for OXTR and 5-HTT Genes," *Journal of Family Psychology* 26 (2012): 431-442.

66 *On one late afternoon in 2007, forty-seven couples entered the unassuming steel-and-concrete buildings of the University of Zurich . . .* Beate Ditzen et al., "Intranasal Oxytocin Increases Positive Communication and Reduces Cortisol Levels During Couple Conflict," *Biological Psychiatry* 65 (2009): 728-731.

67 *It makes us better at reading facial expressions of emotions . . .* —Gregor Domes et al., "Oxytocin improves 'mind-reading' in humans," *Biological Psychiatry* 6 (2007).

67 *It makes us more trusting.* —Michael Kosfeld et al., "Oxytocin increased trust in humans," *Nature* (2005).

67 *It can even make husbands stand further away from pretty women.* —Dirk Scheele et al., "Oxytocin Modulates Social Distance between Males and Females," *Journal of Neuroscience* 32 (2012).

68 *There is evidence that oxytocin has anti-inflammatory properties . . .* —C. Sue Carter, "Oxytocin Pathways and the Evolution of Human Behavior," *Annual Review of Psychology* 65 (2014): 17-39.

69 *. . . some researchers have even dubbed it the "elixir of youth."* —Susan E. Erdman, "Microbes and healthful longevity," *Aging* 8 (2016).

69 *. . . their hearts were in far worse shape, too. Yet these effects could be reversed with simple injections of oxytocin.* —Manal Tabbaa et al., "Neuropeptide Regulation of Social Attachment: The Prairie Vole Model," *Comprehensive Physiology* 7 (2016): 81-104.

70 *Even your success in speed dating may be affected by serotonin.* —Karen Wu et al., "Gender Interacts with Opioid Receptor Polymorphism A118G and Serotonin Receptor Polymorphism–1438 A/G on Speed-Dating Success," *Human Nature* 27 (2016): 244-260.

70 *. . . social isolation makes the levels of the neurotransmitter plummet, which in turn can prompt aggressive behaviours . . .* —Simon N. Young, "The effect of raising and lowering tryptophan levels on human mood and social behaviour," *Philosophical Transactions of the Royal Society* B 368 (2013).

70 *It has even been directly connected to longevity . . .* —Sara Fidalgo, Dobril K. Ivanov and Shona H. Wood, "Serotonin: from top to bottom," *Biogerontology* 14 (2013): 21-45.

70 *One study of Japanese centenarians suggests there may be a link in humans, too.* —Yasuyuki Gondo et al., "Contribution of an affect-associated gene to human longevity: Prevalence of the long-allele genotype of the serotonin transporter-linked gene in Japanese centenarians," *Mechanisms of Ageing and Development* 126 (2005): 1178-1184.

70 *Also unlike oxytocin, it appears that more vasopressin circulating in the body is not necessarily better . . .* —Florina Uzefovsky et al., "Vasopressin selectively impairs emotion recognition in men," *Psychoneuroendocrinology* 37 (2012): 576-580.

71 *It can make rat mothers fiercely protective of their babies . . .* —Oliver J. Bosch and Inga D. Neumann, "Both oxytocin and vasopressin are mediators of maternal care and aggression in rodents: from central release to sites of action," *Hormones and Behavior* 61 (2012): 293-202.

71   *. . . both males and females swap partners left and right.* —Renee C. Firman and Leigh W. Simmons, "Experimental evolution of sperm quality via postcopulatory sexual selection in house mice," *Evolution* 64 (2010): 1245-1256.

71   *Back in the late 1990s, Larry Young and his colleagues at the Atlanta lab . . .* —Larry J. Young et al., "Increased affiliative response to vasopressin in mice expressing the V$_{1a}$ receptor from a monogamous vole," *Nature* 400 (1999): 766-768.

71   *A study of Swedish twins revealed that in men, polymorphisms of one vasopressin gene in particular, called* AVPR1A *. . .* —Hasse Walum et al., "Genetic variation in the vasopressin receptor 1a gene (*AVPR1A*) associates with pair-bonding behavior in humans," *PNAS* 105 (2008): 14153-14156.

72   *In experiments, squirting vasopressin up people's noses has been shown to improve sleep and memory . . .* —Boris Perras et al., "Beneficial Treatment of Age-Related Sleep Disturbances With Prolonged Intranasal Vasopressin," *Journal of Clinical Psychopharmacology* 19 (1999): 28-36.

72   *. . . and to make women more conciliatory and men better at cooperation . . .* —James K. Rilling et al., "Sex differences in the neural and behavioral response to intranasal oxytocin and vasopressin during human social interaction," *Psychoneuroendocrinology* 39 (2014).

72   *When mama rats engage in a lot of skin-to-skin contact with their babies . . .* — S. Kojima et al., "Maternal Contact Differentially Modulates Central and Peripheral Oxytocin in Rat Pups During a Brief Regime of Mother–Pup Interaction that Induces a Filial Huddling Preference," *Journal of Neuroendocrinology* 24 (2012): 831-840.

73   *Mothers and fathers who have high oxytocin are more responsive, more sensitive, and warmer toward their kids . . .* —Ilanit Gordon et al., "Oxytocin and the Development of Parenting in Humans," *Biological Psychiatry* 68 (2010): 377-382.

73   *Massage therapy can boost serotonin by 28 percent and dopamine by 31 percent.* — Tiffany Field et al., "Cortisol decreases and serotonin and dopamine increase following massage therapy," *International Journal of Neuroscience* 10 (2005).

73   *Several studies have shown that orgasms are quite good at raising oxytocin levels in the blood.* —S. Ogawa et al., "Increase in oxytocin secretion at ejaculation in male," Clinical Endocrinology 13 (1980): 95-97 AND W. Blaicher et al., "The role of oxytocin in relation to female sexual arousal," *Gynecologic and Obstetric Investigation* 47 (1999): 125-126.

73   *. . . the more a mother looks at her baby's face, the more oxytocin gets pumped into her body.* —Lane Strathearn et al., "Adult attachment predicts maternal brain and oxytocin response to infant cues," *Neuropsychopharmacology* 34 (2009): 2655-2666.

73   *More remarkable was an experiment published in 2015 in the journal* Science *. . .* —M. Nagasawa et al., "Oxytocin-gaze positive loop and the coevolution of human-dog bonds," *Science* 348 (2015): 333-336.

73   *When little mice are allowed to interact with other little mice in their nest, they grow up to have more oxytocin receptors in specific areas of their brains.* —Igor Branchi et al.,

"Early interactions with mother and peers independently build adult social skills and shape BDNF and oxytocin receptor brain levels," *Psychoneuroendocrinology* 38 (2013): 522-532.

74 *. . . foods containing tryptophan don't increase brain serotonin.* —Simon N. Young, "How to increase serotonin in the human brain without drugs," *Journal of Psychiatry & Neuroscience* 32 (2007): 394-399.

PART TWO: HOW YOUR RELATIONSHIPS AND YOUR MIND CAN PROLONG YOUR LIFE

CHAPTER 4: DITCH GOJI BERRIES

81 *One study done in Mississippi suggested that for every unit increase in BMI . . .* —Jongha Park et al., "Obesity Paradox in End-Stage Kidney Disease Patients," *Progress in Cardiovascular Diseases* 56 (2016): 415-425.

81 *If the illness progresses to a full-blown heart failure . . .* —Jeptha P. Curtis et al., "The Obesity Paradox: Body Mass Index and Outcomes in Patients With Heart Failure," *JAMA* 165 (2005): 55-61.

81 *The obesity paradox has been found in hypertension, in atrial fibrillation (a heart condition) . . .* —Carl J. Lavie et al., "Obesity and Cardiovascular Diseases," *Journal of the American College of Cardiology* 63 (2014).

81 *. . . and in lung-removal surgery.* —L. Tulinský et al., "Obesity paradox in patients undergoing lung lobectomy—myth or reality?" *BMC Surgery* 18 (2018).

81 *People with BMIs between 30 and 35, which is grade one obesity and above normal BMI of 18.5 to 24.9 . . .* —Katherine Flegal et al., Association of All-Cause Mortality With Overweight and Obesity Using Standard Body Mass Index Categories," *JAMA* 309 (2013).

82 *One explanation for such counterintuitive results is that BMI is simply not a good measurement of how extra pounds affect health.* —BMI is calculated by simply dividing a person's weight in kilograms by height in metres squared.

82 *For one, it can sop up toxins.* —Jongha Park et al., "Obesity Paradox in End-Stage Kidney Disease Patients," *Progress in Cardiovascular Diseases* 56 (2016): 415-425.

83 *Here is what he recounted: "you are showing both signs of starvation and of protein poisoning . . ."*—"Vihljalmur Stefansson was called and examined, May 8, 1919," accessed November 27, 2014, https://openlibrary.org/books/OL24661516M/Vihjalmur_Stefansson_was_called_and_examined_May_8_1919_i.e._1920

83 *. . . eating a lot of protein can accelerate the illness, so much so that scientists now advise against such diets in patients with chronic renal disease.* —Adam M. Bernstein, Leo Treyzon and Zhaoping Li, "Are High-Protein, Vegetable-Based Diets Safe for Kidney Function? A Review of the Literature," *Journal of the American Dietetic Association* 107 (2007): 644-650.

83 *Authors of a study that revealed worrisome changes in renal function in young men . . .* —Helga Frank et al., "Effect of short-term high-protein compared with normal-

protein diets on renal hemodynamics and associated variables in healthy young men," *The American Journal of Clinical Nutrition* 90 (2009): 1509-1516.

83 *Very low-carbohydrate diets may elevate the risk of imminent death by as much as 31 percent.* —Hiroshi Noto et al., "Low-Carbohydrate Diets and All-Cause Mortality: A Systematic Review and Meta-Analysis of Observational Studies," *PLOS One* 8 (2013).

84 *A fifty-five-year-old Indian national living in Canada . . .* —Harinder Singh Bedi, Vivek Tewarson and Kamal Negi, "Bleeding risk of dietary supplements: A hidden nightmare for cardiac surgeons," *Indian Heart Journal* 68 (2016): S249-S250.

84 *Each year in the US alone there are an estimated fifty thousand serious adverse events connected to supplement consumption.* —Pieter A. Cohen, "American Roulette—Contaminated Dietary Supplements," *The New England Journal of Medicine* 361 (2009): 1523-1525.

84 *In 2013, as many as 20 percent of cases of drug-induced liver injury were due to herbal and dietary supplements . . .* —Victor J. Navarro et al., "Liver injury from Herbals and Dietary Supplements in the US Drug Induced Liver Injury Network," *Hepatology* 60 (2014): 1399-1408.

85 *First of all, about a quarter of supplements may have contaminants in them . . .* —Antonia C. Novello et al., "Dietary Supplements Balancing Consumer Choice & Safety," *New York State Task Force on Life & the Law*, 2006, accessed July 30, 2019, https://www.health.ny.gov/regulations/task_force/docs/dietary_supplement_safety.pdf

85 *As of 2014, over five hundred supplements have been found to be tainted with pharmaceuticals . . .* —Pieter A. Cohen, "Hazards of Hindsight — Monitoring the Safety of Nutritional Supplements," *New England Journal of Medicine* 370 (2014): 1277-1280.

87 *According to meta-analyses of studies, taking at least 400 IU or more of vitamin E per day can actually shorten your life . . .* —Edgar R. Miller III et al., "Meta-Analysis: High-Dosage Vitamin E Supplementation May Increase All-Cause Mortality," *Annals of Internal Medicine* 142 (2005): 37-46.

87 *. . . and so can beta-carotene supplements and vitamin A.* —Goran Bjelakovic et al., "Antioxidant Supplements to Prevent Mortality," *JAMA* 310 (2013): 1178-1179.

87 *In a study of over eighty thousand American physicians, those who took multivitamin pills had a 7 percent higher risk of dying . . .* —Jorg Muntwyler et al., Vitamin Supplement Use in a Low-Risk Population of US Male Physicians and Subsequent Cardiovascular Mortality," *JAMA Internal Medicine* 162 (2002): 1472-1476.

89 *"The enthusiasm for the health benefits of M. oleifera is in dire contrast with the scarcity of strong experimental and clinical evidence supporting them."* —Majambu Mbikay, "Therapeutic potential of *Moringa oleifera* leaves in chronic hyperglycemia and dyslipidemia: a review," *Frontiers in Pharmacology* (2012).

89 *A 2017 review published in the* Journal of Medicinal Chemistry . . . —Kathryn M. Nelson et al., "The Essential Medicinal Chemistry of Curcumin," *The Journal of Medicinal Chemistry* 60 (2017): 1620-1637.

89 *So far no double-blinded, placebo-controlled clinical trial involving curcumin has been successful.* —ibid.

90 *In one investigation of over 1,700 products available on the British market* . . . —L. Fry, A.M. Madden, R. Fallaize, "An investigation into the nutritional composition and cost of gluten-free versus regular food products in the UK.," *Journal of Human Nutrition and Dietetics* 31 (2018): 108-120.

90 . . . *contain lower amounts of some vitamins.* —Giorgia Vici et al., "Gluten free diet and nutrient deficiencies: A review," *Clinical Nutrition* 35 (2016): 1236-1241.

90 *In one study, blood and urine samples of people on gluten-free diets had 47 percent higher levels of mercury and 80 percent higher levels of arsenic.* —Stephanie L. Raehsler et al., "Accumulation of Heavy Metals in People on a Gluten-Free Diet," *Clinical Gastroenterology and Hepatology* 16 (2018): 244-251.

90 *As a result, epidemiological research shows that people who habitually eat low amounts of gluten tend to have more diabetes* . . . —Geng Zong et al., " Gluten intake and risk of type 2 diabetes in three large prospective cohort studies of US men and women," *Diabetologia* 61 (2018): 2164-2173

90 *One study done in California has shown that vegetarians may live longer than others* . . . —Fraser and Shavlik, Ten Years of Life; Paul N. Appleby et al., "The Oxford Vegetarian Study: an overview," *The American Journal of Clinical Nutrition* 70 (1999): 525s-531s.

90 *Adding three ounces (85 g) of red meat to your daily diet* . . . —An Pan et al., "Red Meat Consumption and Mortality," *Archives of Internal Medicine* 172 (2012).

91 *In one 2014 interview, fashion designer Dame Vivienne Westwood* . . . —Anita Singh, "Vivienne Westwood: People who can't afford organic food should eat less," *The Telegraph,* accessed July 30, 2019, https://www.telegraph.co.uk/news/health/news/11225326/Vivienne-Westwood-People-who-cant-afford-organic-food-should-eat-less.html

91 *Take, for example, a trial in which a group of women consumed either 3.4 ounces (96 g) of organic or conventional tomato purée per day for three weeks* . . . —Alan D Dangour et al., "Nutrition-related health effects of organic foods: a systematic review," *The American Journal of Clinical Nutrition* 92 (2010): 203-210.

91 *Well, in another study that had people eat 1.1 pounds (500 g) of apples a day for almost a month* . . . —ibid.

91 *In a Danish trial, sixteen people ate either a strictly controlled organic diet* . . . —Lisbeth Grinder-Pedersen et al., "Effect of Diets Based on Foods from Conventional versus Organic Production on Intake and Excretion of Flavonoids and Markers of Antioxidative Defense in Humans," *Journal of Agricultural and Food Chemistry* 51 (2003): 5671-5676.

92 . . . *pyrethrum comes out at least as acutely toxic as the infamous synthetic pesticide chlorpyrifos.* —Amanpreet S. Dhillon et al., "Pesticide/Environmental Exposures and Parkinson's Disease in East Texas," *Journal of Agromedicine* 13 (2008): 37-48.

92 *Rotenone, meanwhile, another organic pesticide, ups the risk of Parkinson's disease by as much as eleven times.* —Caroline M. Tanner et al., "Rotenone, Paraquat, and Parkinson's Disease," *Environmental Health Perspectives* 119 (2011): 866-872.

92   *In an interview with the* Washington Post, *Nate Lewis, farm policy director for the Organic Trade Association, commented on organic eating . . .* —Tamar Haspel, "The truth about organic produce and pesticides," *The Washington Post,* accessed July 31, 2019, https://www.washingtonpost.com/lifestyle/food/the-truth-about-organic-produce-and-pesticides/2018/05/18/8294296e-5940-11e8-858f-12becb4d6067_story.html?utm_term=.23d0d9e722d3

93   *That's why the United States Environmental Protection Agency states on its website . . .* —"Food and pesticides," EPA, accessed July 31, 2019, https://www.epa.gov/safepestcontrol/food-and-pesticides

93   *Pesticide applicators from Iowa and North Carolina who regularly deal with certain chemicals have double the risk of lung cancer.* —Matthew R. Bonner et al., "Occupational Exposure to Pesticides and the Incidence of Lung Cancer in the Agricultural Health Study," *Environmental Health Perspectives* 125 (2017).

93   *Applying such products four or more times per year may increase the risk of melanoma by 44 percent.* —Majoriê M. Segatto et al., "Residential and occupational exposure to pesticides may increase risk for cutaneous melanoma: a case–control study conducted in the south of Brazil," *International Journal of Dermatology* 54 (2015): e527-e538.

93   *Some scientists go as far as to argue that synthetic pesticides, just like the natural ones we eat in fruits and vegetables . . .* —Anthony Trewavas and Derek Stewart, "Paradoxical effects of chemicals in the diet on health," *Current Opinion in Plant Biology* 6 (2003): 185-190.

93   *. . . animal research does show that small doses of many supposedly toxic chemicals . . .* —Anthony Trewavas, "A critical assessment of organic farming-and-food assertions with particular respect to the UK and the potential environmental benefits of no-till agriculture," *Crop Protection* 23 (2004).

93   *"Vegetables, fruits, and whole grains should continue to form the central part of the diet . . ."*—Lawrence H. Kushi et al., "American Cancer Society Guidelines on Nutrition and Physical Activity for Cancer Prevention," *ACS Guidelines on Nutrition and Physical Activity for Cancer Prevention* (2012).

94   *Yet in seventeen years of practice in Roseto, the local physician, Dr. Benjamin Falcone . . .* —Stewart Wolf et al., "Roseto, Pennsylvania 25 Years Later—Highlights of a Medical and Sociological Survey," *Transactions of the American Clinical and Climatological Association* 100 (1989).

95   *In the words of one Rosetan housewife . . .* —Harrington, Anne. *The Cure Within: A History of Mind-Body Medicine* (New York: W.W. Norton & Company: 2008), 180.

96   *A happy marriage equals a 49 percent lower mortality risk.* —Julianne Holt-Lunstad, David A. Sbarra and Theodore F. Robles, "Advancing Social Connection as a Public Health Priority in the United States," *American Psychologist* 72 (2017).

96   *Living with someone, even just a roommate, as opposed to living alone . . .* —Julianne Holt-Lunstad, Timothy B. Smith and J. Bradley Layton, "Social Relationships and Mortality Risk: A Meta-analytic Review," *PLOS Medicine* (2010) AND Julianne Holt-Lunstad, David A. Sbarra and Theodore F. Robles, "Advancing

Social Connection as a Public Health Priority in the United States," *American Psychologist* 72 (2017).

96 *Having a large network of friends: 45 percent.* —Julianne Holt-Lunstad, David A. Sbarra and Theodore F. Robles, "Advancing Social Connection as a Public Health Priority in the United States," *American Psychologist* 72 (2017).

97 *. . . Roseto effect, you would get a whopping 65 percent reduction in mortality.* —Julianne Holt-Lunstad, Timothy B. Smith and J. Bradley Layton, "Social Relationships and Mortality Risk: A Meta-analytic Review," *PLOS Medicine* (2010).

97 *A study done in Singapore showed that using a Fitbit does not lead to improved health or fitness.* —Eric A. Finkelstein et al., "Effectiveness of activity trackers with and without incentives to increase physical activity (TRIPPA): a randomised controlled trial," *The Lancet* 4 (2016): 983-995.

97 *Even more troubling was another trial in which wearing a fitness tracker actually led to a slower weight loss.* —John M. Jakicic et al., "Effect of Wearable Technology Combined With a Lifestyle Intervention on Long-term Weight Loss," *JAMA* 316 (2016): 1161-1171.

97 *. . . you can push your risk of death down by about 66 percent.* —Martin Loef and Harald Walach, "The combined effects of hsealthy lifestyle behaviors on all cause mortality: A systematic review and meta-analysis," *Preventive Medicine* 55 (2012): 163-170.

Table 1a

100 *Whole grain intake—3 servings/day: –23%* —Lyn M Steffen et al., "Associations of whole-grain, refined-grain, and fruit and vegetable consumption with risks of all-cause mortality and incident coronary artery disease and ischemic stroke: the Atherosclerosis Risk in Communities (ARIC) Study," *The American Journal of Clinical Nutrition* 78 (2003): 383-390.

100 *Cruciferous vegetables intake—minimum 5.8 oz/day: –20%* —"Cruciferous vegetable consumption is associated with a reduced risk of total and cardiovascular disease mortality," *The American Journal of Clinical Nutrition* 94 (2011): 240–246.

Table 1b

100 *Feeling you have others you can count on for support: –35%* —Julianne Holt-Lunstad, Timothy B. Smith and J. Bradley Layton, "Social Relationships and Mortality Risk: A Meta-analytic Review," *PLOS Medicine* (2010).

100 *Extraversion: –24%* —Eileen K. Graham et al., "Personality Predicts Mortality Risk: An Integrative Data Analysis of 15 International Longitudinal Studies," *Journal of Research in Personality* (2017).

100 *Agreeableness: –20%* —ibid.

100 *Having a purpose in life: –17%* —Randy Cohen, Chirag Bavishi and Alan Rozanski, "Purpose in Life and Its Relationship to All-Cause Mortality and Cardiovascular Events: A Meta-Analysis," *Psychosomatic Medicine* 78 (2016).

Table 2a

101 *Red meat intake: +29%* —Susanna C. Larsson and Nicola Orsini, "Red Meat and Processed Meat Consumption and All-Cause Mortality: A Meta-Analysis," *American Journal of Epidemiology* 179 (2014): 282-289.

101 *Obesity, grade 2 and 3: +29%* —Katherine M. Flegal et al., "Association of All-Cause Mortality With Overweight and Obesity Using Standard Body Mass Index Categories, a Systematic Review and Meta-analysis," *JAMA* 309 (2013): 71-82.

101 *Vitamin A supplementation: +16%* —Goran Bjelakovic et al., "Mortality in Randomized Trials of Antioxidant Supplements for Primary and Secondary Prevention. Systematic Review and Meta-analysis," *JAMA* 297 (2007): 842-857.

101 *Beta-carotene supplementation: +7%* —ibid.

Table 2b

101 *Pessimism: +14%* —Hilary A. Tindle et al., "Optimism, Cynical Hostility, and Incident Coronary Heart Disease and Mortality in the Women's Health Initiative," *Circulation* 120 (2009): 656-662.

101 *Unhappiness: +14%* —Elizabeth M. Lawrence, Richard G. Rogers and Tim Wadsworth, "Happiness and Longevity in the United States," *Social Science & Medicine* 145 (2015): 115-119.

101 *Neuroticism: +14%* —Páraic S. O'Súilleabháin and Brian M.Hughes, "Neuroticism predicts all-cause mortality over 19-years: The moderating effects on functional status, and the angiotensin-converting enzyme," *Journal of Psychosomatic Research* 110 (2018): 32-37.

CHAPTER 5: THE GNAWING PARASITE OF LONELINESS

104 *A large, high-quality study conducted in Alameda County, California . . .* —Lisa Berkman and S. Leonard Syme, "Social Networks, Host Resistance, and Mortality: a Nine-Year Follow-up Study of Alameda County Residents," *American Journal of Epidemiology* 109 (1979)

104 *It's been shown over and over that people of any age who have poor social relations . . .* —N.K. Valtorta et al., "Loneliness and social isolation as risk factors for coronary heart disease and stroke: systematic review and meta-analysis of longitudinal observational studies," *Heart* (2016) AND G.F. Giesbrecht et al., "The buffering effect of social support on hypothalamic-pituitary-adrenal axis function during pregnancy," *Psychosomatic Medicine* 75 (2013): 856-862.

105 *. . . compared to loners, people who are surrounded by caring others are over three times as likely to listen to their doctors and take their pills as prescribed.* —M. Robin DiMatteo, "Social Support and Patient Adherence to Medical Treatment: A Meta-Analysis," *Health Psychology* 23 (2004): 207-218.

105 *Imagine over three hundred people coming into a research lab and getting voluntarily infected with cold viruses squirted directly into their nostrils . . .* —Sheldon Cohen et al., "Sociability and Susceptibility to the Common Cold," *Psychological Science* 14 (2003).

106 *"I would stand in front of the window looking out over the neighborhood . . ."* —The Loneliness Project, accessed May 27, 2018, http://thelonelinessproject.org

107 *One 2015 meta-analysis of studies established that while objective social isolation may increase the risk of death by 29 percent . . .* —Julianne Holt-Lunstad and Timothy B. Smith, "Loneliness and Social Isolation as Risk Factors for Mortality: A Meta-Analytic Review," *Perspectives on Psychological Science* 10 (2015): 227-237.

108 *If you add up multiple indicators of social support, objective and subjective . . .* —Julianne Holt-Lunstad, Timothy B. Smith and J. Bradley Layton, "Social Relationships and Mortality Risk: A Meta-analytic Review," *PLOS Medicine* (2010).

109 *In his lab studies, Cacioppo found that lonely people experience more fragmented and restless sleep . . .* —John Cacioppo et al., "Do lonely days invade the nights? Potential social modulation of sleep efficiency," *Psychological Science* 13 (2002): 385–388.

112 *In one experiment, researchers asked volunteers to play* Cyberball *while inside a magnetic resonance imaging scanner.* —N.I. Eisenberger, M.D. Lieberman and K.D. Williams, "Does rejection hurt? An fMRI study of social exclusion," *Science* 302 (2003): 290-292.

113 *Carriers of the GG variant of the oxytocin receptor gene* rs53576 *feel more gloom . . .* —Robyn J. McQuaid et al., "Distress of ostracism: oxytocin receptor gene polymorphism confers sensitivity to social exclusion," *Social Cognitive and Affective Neuroscience* 10 (2015).

113 *In one fascinating but disturbing study, scientists collected reports on loneliness from 181 people.* —Turhan Canli et al., "Loneliness 5 years ante-mortem is associated with disease-related differential gene expression in postmortem dorsolateral prefrontal cortex," *Translational Psychiatry* 8 (2018).

114 *. . . two Yale University researchers calculated that people who consider themselves socially isolated take more warm baths and showers.* —John A. Bargh and Idit Shalev, "The Substitutability of Physical and Social Warmth in Daily Life," *Emotion* 12 (2012): 154-162.

114 *In one experiment, researchers approached dozens of people who were lunching at a food court . . .* —Andrew W. Perkins, Jeff Rotman and Seung Hwan (Mark) Lee, "Embodied Cognition and Social Consumption: Self- Regulating Temperature Through Social Products and Behaviors," *Journal of Consumer Psychology* 24 (2014): 234-240.

114 *Such recollections can make people estimate the room temperature as higher than it really is by as much as 3.6 degrees Fahrenheit (2.0°C.).* —Aleksandra Szymkow et al., "Warmer Hearts, Warmer Rooms How Positive Communal Traits Increase Estimates of Ambient Temperature," *Social Psychology* 44 (2013): 167-176.

115 *Holding a steaming drink in their hands makes people more trusting and "warm" toward fellow humans.* —Lawrence E. Williams and John A. Bargh, "Experiencing Physical Warmth Promotes Interpersonal Warmth," *Science* 322 (2008).

115 *For many animals, huddling allows them to save precious energy resources.* —Hans IJzerman et al., "A theory of social thermoregulation in human primates," *Frontiers in Psychology* (2015).

117 *In a laboratory room at the University of Central Lancashire, UK . . .* —Munirah Bangee et al., "Loneliness and attention to social threat in young adults: Findings from an eye tracker study," *Personality and Individual Differences* 63 (2014).

119 *"Is it literally true that everybody hates me? No? Then why do I keep saying this to myself?"* —Cacioppo, Johan and William Patrick. *Loneliness: Human Nature*

and the Need for Social Connection (New York: W.W. Norton & Company: 2008), 236.

119 . . . *studies show that if people are hypnotized and their thoughts are redirected toward feelings of social connection* . . . —John T. Cacioppo et al., "Loneliness within a nomological net: An evolutionary perspective," *Journal of Research in Personality* 40 (2006): 1054-1085.

119 *In one experiment conducted in Switzerland and published in the prestigious journal of the National Academy of Sciences* . . . —Katrin H. Preller et al., "Effects of serotonin 2A/1A receptor stimulation on social exclusion processing," *PNAS* 113 (2016): 5119-5124.

CHAPTER 6: FRIENDS WITH (LONGEVITY) BENEFITS

122 *Research shows that married people have lower risks of heart issues, cancer, and Alzheimer's disease.* —C. Helmer et al., "Marital Status and Risk of Alzheimer's Disease," *Neurology* 53 (1999).

122 *They even sleep more soundly* . . . —Jen-Hao Chen, Linda J. Waite and Diane S. Lauderdale, "Marriage, Relationship Quality, and Sleep among U.S. Older Adults," *Journal of Health and Social Behavior* 56 (2015).

122 . . . *and respond better to flu vaccines.* —Anna C.Phillips et al., "Bereavement and marriage are associated with antibody response to influenza vaccination in the elderly," *Brain, Behavior, and Immunity* 20 (2006): 279-289.

122 *If a married person does have a heart attack requiring coronary artery bypass grafting* . . . —Kathleen B. King and Harry T. Reis, "Marriage and long-term survival after coronary artery bypass grafting," *Health Psychology* 31 (2012): 55-62.

122 *When researchers followed over 700,000 patients with several different types of cancer* . . . —Ayal A. Aizer et al., "Marital Status and Survival in Patients With Cancer," *Journal of Clinical Oncology* 31 (2013): 3869-3876.

122 *In one large sample, not being married meant even three times the risk of death for men, and a risk of 20 percent higher for women.* —Richard G. Rogers, "Marriage, Sex, and Mortality," *Journal of Marriage and Family* 57 (1995):515-526.

123 . . . *the most dangerous period is the first week—the risk of dying from natural causes doubles for them.* —J. Kaprio, M. Koskenvuo and H. Rita, "Mortality after bereavement: a prospective study of 95,647 widowed persons," *American Journal of Public Health* (1987).

125 *In a Finnish study published in 2015, those who cohabited without "putting a ring on it"* . . . —Fanny Kilpi et al., "Living arrangements as determinants of myocardial infarction incidence and survival: A prospective register study of over 300,000 Finnish men and women," *Social Science & Medicine* 133 (2015).

126 *For both spouses, low marital satisfaction has been linked to physiological processes* . . . —Sarah C. E. Stanton and Lorne Campbell, "Psychological and Physiological Predictors of Health in Romantic Relationships: An Attachment Perspective," *Journal of Personality* 82 (2014).

126 *Happily married women, meanwhile, are three times less likely to develop the metabolic syndrome* . . . —Janice K. Kiecolt-Glaser et al., "Marital Discord, Past Depression, and Metabolic Responses to High-Fat Meals: Interpersonal Pathways to Obesity," *Psychoneuroendocrinology* 52 (2015): 239-250.

126 *Two Chinese studies have found that arranged marriages don't bring the same levels of well-being* . . . —Keera Allendorf, "Determinants of Marital Quality in an Arranged Marriage Society," *Social Science Research* 42 (2013): 59-70.

127 *In one rather unpleasant experiment, a few dozen married couples were invited into a lab* . . . —Jean-Philippe Gouin et al., "Marital Behavior, Oxytocin, Vasopressin, and Wound Healing," *Psychoneuroendocrinology* 35 (2010): 1082-1090.

127 *Romantic couples tend to synchronize their blood pressure, cortisol levels, pulse, heart rate, finger temperature, and electrical activity in the chest.* —Adela C. Timmons, Gayla Margolin, and Darby E. Saxbe, "Physiological Linkage in Couples and its Implications for Individual and Interpersonal Functioning: A Literature Review," *Journal of Family Psychology* 29 (2015): 720–731.

128 *Being divorced means about 30 percent higher risk of death* . . . —Eran Shor et al., "Meta-analysis of Marital Dissolution and Mortality: Reevaluating the Intersection of Gender and Age," *Social Science & Medicine* 75 (2012).

129 *Certainly for the Betars, named the "longest-married couple in America," good marriage did seem to pair with good health* . . . — Simmy Richman, "John Betar: Syrian refugee and wife Ann become 'longest married couple in America' after being together for 83 years," *The Independent*, accessed https://www.independent.co.uk/voices/john-betar-syrian-refugee-and-wife-ann-become-longest-married-couple-in-america-after-being-together-a6872806.html

129 *"We never hold grudges. Most arguments are about food," John said.* —Kashmira Gander, "John and Ann Betar: Couple Married for 83 Years Give Relationship Advice on Twitter," *The Independent*, accessed August 1, 2019, https://www.independent.co.uk/life-style/love-sex/john-and-ann-betar-couple-married-for-83-years-give-relationship-advice-on-twitter-a6876806.html

129 *"We are not arguing; we are listening. And we've always listened," she said.* —Lindsey Smith, "America's 'Longest-Married Couple' Celebrates Historic 85th Wedding Anniversary," Little Things, accessed August 1, 2019, https://www.littlethings.com/longest-married-couple-85-years/

129 *. . . it was possible to predict whether a couple would stay married over the next fourteen years with 93 percent accuracy* . . . —John Mordechai Gottman and Robert Wayne Levenson, "The Timing of Divorce: Predicting When a Couple Will Divorce Over a 14-Year Period," *Journal of Marriage and Family* 62 (2000): 737-745.

130 *The couples who volunteered for the study had to discuss a conflict topic for twenty minutes* . . . —Janice K. Kiecolt-Glaser et al., "Marital Discord, Past Depression, and Metabolic Responses to High-Fat Meals: Interpersonal Pathways to Obesity," *Psychoneuroendocrinology* 52 (2015): 239-250.

132   . . . *research also shows that doing thrilling activities with someone you are attracted to fools your body on physiological level.* —Donald Dutton and Arthur Aron, "Some evidence for heightened sexual attraction under conditions of high anxiety," *Journal of Personality and Social Psychology* 30 (1974): 510-517.

133   . . . *even fruit flies have shorter lives if they don't have BFFs.* —Hongyu Ruan and Chun-Fang Wu,"Social interaction-mediated lifespan extension of Drosophila Cu/Zn superoxide dismutase mutants," *PNAS* 105 (2008): 7506–7510.

134   *Mice don't take well to seclusion, either.* —Navita Kaushal et al., "Socially Isolated Mice Exhibit a Blunted Homeostatic Sleep Response to Acute Sleep Deprivation Compared to Socially Paired Mice," *Brain Research* 1454 (2012): 65-79.

134   *In one Japanese study, older men who met their friends less than a few times per year had 30 percent higher risk of dying . . .* —Jun Aida et al., "Assessing the association between all-cause mortality and multiple aspects of individual social capital among the older Japanese," *BMC Public Health* 11 (2011).

134   *When scientists studied elderly twins in Denmark, they also discovered that frequent contact with friends meant lower risk . . .* —Domenica Rasulo, Kaare Christensen and Cecilia Tomassini, "The Influence of Social Relations on Mortality in Later Life: A Study on Elderly Danish Twins," *The Gerontologist* 45 (2005): 601-608.

134   *The impact of friendship on longevity is so large that in many studies it overshadows the impact of how often you meet with your relatives . . .* —ibid.

135   *A Dutch study showed, for example, that each additional contact in your network . . .* —Lea Ellwardt et al,"Personal Networks and Mortality Risk in Older Adults: A Twenty-Year Longitudinal Study," *PLOS One* (2015).

136   . . . *for instance, women have on average 3.8 friends in their "hair-care" networks . . .* —Kazuyoshi Sugawara, "Spatial Proximity and Bodily Contact among the Central Kalahari San," *African Study Monograph* (1984).

137   . . . *even though real-life friendships boosted self-reported health, Facebook ones did not.* —Maria Luisa Lima et al., "All You Need Is Facebook Friends? Associations between Online and Face-to-Face Friendships and Health," *Frontiers in Psychology* (2017).

137   *In yet another, high proportions of Facebook friends to offline ones meant higher levels of social isolation and loneliness.* —Pamara Chang et al., "Age Differences in Online Social Networking: Extending Socioemotional Selectivity Theory to Social Network Sites," *Journal of Broadcasting & Electronic Media* 59 (2015): 221-239.

137   *Other research reveals that hearing your mom's reassuring words on the phone causes a larger oxytocin release . . .* —Leslie J. Seltzer et al., "Instant messages vs. speech: hormones and why we still need to hear each other," *Evolution and Human Behavior* 33 (2012): 42–45.

139   *In a 2012* New York Times *article that went viral . . .* —Alex Williams, "Why Is It Hard to Make Friends Over 30?" *The New York Times*, accessed August 1, 2019, https://www.nytimes.com/2012/07/15/fashion/the-challenge-of-making-friends-as-an-adult.html

140 *A study published in the prestigious journal PNAS showed that friends resemble each other on a genotypic level . . .* —James H. Fowler, Jaime E. Settle and Nicholas A. Christakis, "Correlated genotypes in friendship networks," *PNAS* 108 (2011): 1993-1997.

140 *Police trainees, for example, are more likely to become buddies with other trainees whose last names start with the same letter.* —M.W. Segal, "Alphabet and attraction: An unobtrusive measure of the effect of propinquity in field setting," *Journal of Personality and Social Psychology* 30 (1974): 654–657.

140 *Among university students, those who live in apartments without ensuite bathrooms tend to have stronger interpersonal bonds with their roommates.* —Matthew J. Easterbrook and Vivian L. Vignoles, "When friendship formation goes down the toilet: Design features of shared accommodation influence interpersonal bonds and well-being," *British Journal of Social Psychology* 54 (2015): 125-139.

141 *Studies show that self-disclosure brings people closer together.* —Kelly Campbell, Nicole Holderness and Matt Riggs, "Friendship chemistry: An examination of underlying factors," *Journal of Social Sciences* 52 (2015): 239–247.

142 *Among the elderly of Chicago, for instance, a high level of extraversion meant a 21 percent lower risk of death . . .* —S. Robert et al., "Neuroticism, Extraversion, and Mortality in a Defined Population of Older Persons," *Psychosomatic Medicine* 67 (2005): 841-845.

142 *. . . similar findings came from Japan and Sweden.* —Benjamin P. Chapman, Brent Roberts and Paul Duberstein, "Personality and Longevity: Knowns, Unknowns, and Implications for Public Health and Personalized Medicine," *Journal of Aging Research* (2011).

142 *. . . in one of his studies, Robin Dunbar has found that even though extroverts tend to have more friends, the quality of their relationships isn't necessarily any better than that of introverts.* —Thomas V. Pollet, Sam G. B. Roberts and Robin I. M. Dunbar, "Extraverts Have Larger Social Network Layers But Do Not Feel Emotionally Closer to Individuals at Any Layer," *Journal of Individual Differences* 32 (2011): 161-169.

CHAPTER 7: CHAMELEONS LIVE LONG

145 *"Most subjects typically assume a hunched position in a corner of the bottom of the apparatus . . ."* —Blum, Deborah. *Love at Goon Park: Harry Harlow and the Science of Affection* (New York: Basic Books, 2002).

147 *. . . securely attached babies grow up to be more empathetic, helpful preschoolers who are surrounded by friends.* —Roberta Kestenbaum, Ellen A. Farber and L. Alan Sroufe, "Individual differences in empathy among preschoolers: Relation to attachment history," *New Directions for Child and Adolescent Development* 44 (1989): 51-64.

147 *As preteens, they are more popular and socially competent.* —J. Elicker, M. Englund and L.A. Sroufe, "Predicting peer competence and peer relations in childhood from early parent–child relationships," in *Family–Peer Relationships: Modes of Linkage*, eds. R. D. Parke and G. W. Ladd (Hillsdale, NJ: Lawrence Erlbaum Associates, 1992), 77-106.

148 *Functional magnetic resonance imaging studies show that when people with avoidant attachment style meet their friends . . .* —Pascal Vrtička et al., "Individual attachment style modulates human amygdala and striatum activation during social appraisal," *PLOS One* (2008).

148 *In one recent study, adults with more attachment anxiety dealt less well with a virus that can cause mononucleosis.* —Christopher P. Fagundes et al., "Attachment anxiety is related to Epstein–Barr virus latency," *Brain, Behavior, and Immunity* 41 (2014): 232–238.

148 *. . . those who are anxiously attached have more strokes and heart attacks, higher blood pressure, and more ulcers.* —Lisa M. Jaremka et al., "Attachment Anxiety is Linked to Alterations in Cortisol Production and Cellular Immunity," *Psychological Science* 24 (2013).

148 *They also suffer more often from medically unexplained musculoskeletal pain.* —Corinna Schroeter et al., "Attachment, Symptom Severity, and Depression in Medically Unexplained Musculoskeletal Pain and Osteoarthritis: A Cross-Sectional Study," *PLOS One* (2015).

148 *. . . those who agree with statements such as, "I find it difficult to allow myself to depend on romantic partners" . . .* —Charlotte Krahé et al., "Attachment style moderates partner presence effects on pain: a laser-evoked potentials study," *Social Cognitive and Affective Neuroscience* 10 (2015): 1030-1037.

148 *In one study, people with high attachment anxiety had 22 percent fewer CD3+CD8+ cytotoxic T cells than those with lower attachment anxiety.* —Lisa M. Jaremka et al., "Attachment Anxiety is Linked to Alterations in Cortisol Production and Cellular Immunity," *Psychological Science* 24 (2013).

149 *. . . it may be linked to eating disorders, and binge eating in particular.* —Hilary Maxwell et al., "Change in attachment insecurity is related to improved outcomes 1-year post group therapy in women with binge eating disorder," *Psychotherapy* 51 (2014): 57-65.

149 *Research shows that people who are securely attached are happier with their friendships, fight less with their loved ones, and are less likely to end up divorced.* —R. Chris Fraley et al., "Interpersonal and Genetic Origins of Adult Attachment Styles: A Longitudinal Study from Infancy to Early Adulthood," *Journal of Personality and Social Psychology* 104 (2013).

149 *And even if they have as many friends as others do, they are often quite negative about the support they are getting.* —Sarah C. E. Stanton and Lorne Campbell, "Psychological and Physiological Predictors of Health in Romantic Relationships: An Attachment Perspective," *Journal of Personality* 82 (2014).

150 *The scientists behind the meta-analysis point out that smartphones and internet may be to blame . . .* —Sara H. Konrath et al., "Changes in Adult Attachment Styles in American College Students Over Time: A Meta-Analysis," *Personality and Social Psychology Review* 18 (2014).

151 *Research suggests that as little as six weeks of intensive therapy can boost security of attachment . . .* —Jacqueline L. Kinley and Sandra M. Reyno, "Attachment Style

Changes Following Intensive Short-term Group Psychotherapy," *International Journal of Group Psychotherapy* 63 (2013).

152 *Frans de Waal, a renowned Dutch primatologist, believes that mood contagion evolved . . .* —de Waal, Frans. *The Age of Empathy: Nature's Lessons for a Kinder Society* (New York: Broadway Books, 2009).

153 *In one of his speeches, former president Barack Obama noted that "we live in a culture that discourages empathy."* —"Obama to Graduates: Cultivate Empathy," Northwestern University, accessed August 1, 2019, https://www.northwestern.edu/newscenter/stories/2006/06/barack.html

153 *. . . studies confirm that those who are financially very well off tend to score low on empathy.* —Paul K. Piff et al., "Higher social class predicts increased unethical behavior," *PNAS* 109 (2012): 4086-4091.

153 *In research conducted at Michigan State University, the US ranked seventh from the top among sixty-three countries . . .* —William J. Chopik, Ed O'Brien and Sara H. Konrath, "Differences in Empathic Concern and Perspective Taking Across 63 Countries," *Journal of Cross-Cultural Psychology* 48 (2017): 23-38.

153 *. . . two-year-old girls showing more concern for people in distress than do boys of the same age.* —de Waal, Frans. *The Age of Empathy: Nature's Lessons for a Kinder Society* (New York: Broadway Books, 2009), 259.

154 *In a study of six- to eight-year-olds that followed such a procedure, the most "outward looking" kids . . .* —Emma Chapman et al., "Fetal testosterone and empathy: Evidence from the Empathy Quotient (EQ) and the 'Reading the Mind in the Eyes' Test," *Social Neuroscience* (2006): 135-148.

154 *Take a teenager, measure their empathy levels, and you will be able to predict how socially well-integrated they will be . . .* —Mathias Allemand, Andrea E. Steiger and Helmut A. Fend, "Empathy Development in Adolescence Predicts Social Competencies in Adulthood," *Journal of Personality* 83 (2015): 229-241.

156 *It works for children, resident physicians, and sex offenders.* —Colin Arthur Wastell, David Cairns and Helen Haywood, "Empathy training, sex offenders and re-offending," *Journal of Sexual Aggression* 15 (2009).

156 *"When I took the bandages off, my skin was all infected because of acne and ingrowing hairs," he told the* Telegraph. —Anne Billson, "The Wonderfully Mad World of Nicolas Cage," *The Telegraph*, accessed August 1, 2019, https://www.telegraph.co.uk/culture/film/10155965/The-wonderfully-mad-world-of-Nicolas-Cage.html

157 *In one experiment, men scored much worse than women on understanding emotion until the researchers offered to pay them for their effort. . .* —Kristi Klein and Sara Hodges, "Gender Differences, Motivation, and Empathic Accuracy: When it Pays to Understand," *Personality and Social Psychology Bulletin* 27 (2001).

157 *In case you are prone to taking acetaminophen pills such as Tylenol . . .* —Dominik Mischkowski, Jennifer Crocker and Baldwin M. Way, "From painkiller to empathy killer: acetaminophen (paracetamol) reduces empathy for pain," *Social Cognitive and Affective Neuroscience* 11 (2016): 1345–1353.

158 *In one of his experiments, simple disco dancing . . .* —Bronwyn Tarr, Jacques Launay and Robin I.M. Dunbar, "Silent disco: dancing in synchrony leads to elevated pain thresholds and social closeness," *Evolution and Human Behavior* 37 (2016): 343–349.

159 *Singing in a choir causes release of endorphins, natural painkillers . . .* —Daniel Weinstein et al., "Singing and social bonding: changes in connectivity and pain threshold as a function of group size," *Evolution and Human Behavior* 37 (2016): 152-158.

159 *Rowing in a group, as compared to rowing alone . . .* —Emma E. A. Cohen et al., "Rowers' high: behavioural synchrony is correlated with elevated pain thresholds," *Biology Letters* 6 (2010): 106-108.

159 *Even tapping your fingers in rhythm with a partner works, promoting warm feelings of togetherness.* —P. Valdesolo and D. Desteno, "Synchrony and the social tuning of compassion," *Emotion* 11 (2011): 262-266.

160 *We humans are so sensitive to synchrony that even fourteen-month-old babies . . .* —Bahar Tunçgenç, Emma Cohen and Christine Fawcett, "Rock With Me: The Role of Movement Synchrony in Infants' Social and Nonsocial Choices," *Child Development* 86 (2015): 976-984.

161 *Synchrony is so powerful, in fact, that coordinating your actions with a complete stranger . . .* —L.J. Martin et al., "Reducing social stress elicits emotional contagion of pain in mouse and human strangers," *Current Biology* 25 (2015): 326-332.

161 *Laughing with others can also work as social grooming, and studies show that it elevates pain thresholds . . .* —Sandra Manninen et al., "Social Laughter Triggers Endogenous Opioid Release in Humans," *Journal of Neuroscience* 37 (2017): 6125-6131.

162 *In one experiment people were presented with a pile of pictures—individual portraits of husbands and wives . . .* —R. B. Zajonc et al., "Convergence in the physical appearance of spouses," *Motivation and Emotion* 11 (1987): 335-346.

162 *Like empathy, mimicry makes us more pro-social, boosts trust, and keeps our blood cortisol low.* —Tanya L. Chartrand and Jessica L. Lakin, "The Antecedents and Consequences of Human Behavioral Mimicry," *Annual Review of Psychology* 64 (2013): 285-308.

162 *. . . and studies show that this process malfunctions in people who get Botox injections.* —Joshua Ian Davis et al., "The Effects of BOTOX® Injections on Emotional Experience," *Emotion* 10 (2010): 433–440.

CHAPTER 8: HELPING OTHERS HELPS YOUR HEALTH

165 *"It was some crazy strength," she recalled later, in an interview for a local Virginia radio station.* —Michael Morrow, "Teenager uses 'superhuman strength' to lift burning truck off dad and save family," News Corp Australia Network, accessed August 2, 2019, https://www.news.com.au/world/north-america/teenager-uses-superhuman-strength-to-lift-burning-truck-off-dad-and-save-family/news-story/9b85e3f96547950c8da3af34c8ee2619

166 *The first inkling that caregiving improves fitness came, unexpectedly, from a 1950s study of housewives.* —Phyllis Moen, Donna Dempster-McClain and Robin M. Williams, Jr., "Successful Aging: A Life-Course Perspective on Women's Multiple Roles and Health," *American Journal of Sociology* 97 (1992).

166 *What's more, volunteers may have 29 percent lower risk of high blood glucose . . .* —Jeffrey A. Burr, Sae Hwang Han and Jane L. Tavares, "Volunteering and Cardiovascular Disease Risk: Does Helping Others Get 'Under the Skin?'" *The Gerontologist* 56 (2016): 937-947.

166 *. . . about 17 percent lower risk of high inflammation levels.* —ibid.

167 *. . . and spend 38 percent fewer nights in hospitals than do people who shy from involvement in charities.* —Eric S. Kim and Sara H. Konrath, "Volunteering is Prospectively Associated with Health Care Use Among Older Adults," *Social Science & Medicine* 149 (2016): 122-129.

167 *In 1961, Michio Ikai of the University of Tokyo and Arthur Steinhaus of George Williams College, Illinois . . .* —Michio Ikai and Arthur Steinhaus, "Some factors modifying the expression of human strength," *Journal of Applied Psychology* 16 (1961).

168 *"People willfully suppress knowledge most have had since childhood, which is that animals do have feelings . . .* —de Waal, Frans. *The Age of Empathy: Nature's Lessons for a Kinder Society* (New York: Broadway Books, 2009), 497.

168 *Rats, for instance, will jailbreak their mates out of their cages . . .* —Inbal Ben-Ami Bartal, Jean Decety and Peggy Mason, "Helping a cagemate in need: empathy and pro-social behavior in rats," *Science* 334 (2011): 1427-1430.

169 *Jim Jefferies, an Australian comedian, once summed up the experience of parenthood in the following way . . .* —Bare, Jim Jefferies, directed by Shannon Hartman, 2014, Netflix, accessed August 8, 2019, https://www.netflix.com/watch/80002621?trackId=13752289&tctx=0%2C0%2Cf6a6e1a7754334028ad220ae599e23f5419d06c7%3A316a4f16246224c4656e5f79e39d124069d1b94c%2C%2C

169 *For elderly human volunteers, caring for infants reduces cortisol levels in the saliva . . .* —Tiffany M. Field et al., "Elder Retired Volunteers Benefit From Giving Massage Therapy to Infants," *Journal of Applied Gerontology* 17 (1998): 229-239.

169 *In general, the more stress people experience in their daily lives, the more beneficial influence helping others exerts on their cortisol.* —Sae Hwang Han, Kyungmin Kim and Jeffrey A. Burr, "Stress-buffering effects of volunteering on salivary cortisol: Results from a daily diary study," *Social Science & Medicine* 201 (2018): 1200-126.

170 *. . . people with damaged amygdalae tend to be do-gooders more often than the rest of us.* —Tristen K. Inagaki, "Neural mechanisms of the link between giving social support and health," *Annals of the New York Academy of Sciences* 1428 (2018): 33-50.

170 *Show parents a photo of their baby and their fear centres quiet down like a newborn with a pacifier.* —ibid.

170 *When people engage in activities that make them experience compassion, the activity of their vagus goes up, too. . .* —Elizabeth B. Raposa, Holly B. Laws and Emily B.

Ansell, "Prosocial Behavior Mitigates the Negative Effects of Stress in Everyday Life," *Clinical Psychological Science* 4 (2016): 691–698.

171 *People who frequently volunteer have lower levels of C-reactive protein . . .* —Jeffrey A. Burr, Sae Hwang Han and Jane L. Tavares, "Volunteering and Cardiovascular Disease Risk: Does Helping Others Get "Under the Skin?" *The Gerontologist* 56 (2016): 937-947.

171 *At one public high school in western Canada, students were divided into two groups.* —Hannah M. C. Schreier, Kimberly A. Schonert-Reichl and Edith Chen, "Effect of Volunteering on Risk Factors for Cardiovascular Disease in Adolescents: A Randomized Controlled Trial," *JAMA Pediatrics* 167 (2013): 327-332.

172 *In one experiment, Aknin and her colleagues handed volunteers either a $5 bill or a $20 bill . . .* —Elizabeth W. Dunn, Lara B. Aknin and Michael I. Norton, "Prosocial Spending and Happiness: Using Money to Benefit Others Pays Off," *Current Directions in Psychological Science* 23 (2014): 41-47.

173 *When Aknin analyzed pro-social spending across the globe . . .* —Lara B. Aknin et al., "Prosocial Spending and Well-Being: Cross-Cultural Evidence for a Psychological Universal," *Journal of Personality and Social Psychology* 104 (2013): 635-652.

173 *The gains can be as varied as better sleep, better hearing, stronger muscles, and lower blood pressure.* —ibid.

173 *When seniors suffering from hypertension were handed $40 per week for three consecutive weeks to either spend on themselves or on someone else . . .* —Ashley V. Whillans et al., "Is spending money on others good for your heart?" *Health Psychology* 35 (2016): 574-583.

173 *In one such experiment, scientists stopped passersby near a subway station in Boston asking if they'd like to try their muscles with a five-pound weight.* —Kurt Gray, "Moral Transformation: Good and Evil Turn the Weak Into the Mighty," *Social Psychological and Personality Science* 1 (2010): 253-258.

174 *Indeed, a widely cited study from 1999 showed that those who reported strain from caring for their disabled spouses . . .* —Richard Schulz and Scott R. Beach, "Caregiving as a Risk Factor for Mortality:" The Caregiver Health Effects Study," *JAMA* 282 (1999): 2215-2219.

174 *In one such analysis, scientists carefully matched over 3,500 family caregivers with more than 3,500 people who didn't nurse anyone . . .* —David L. Roth et al., "Family Caregiving and All-Cause Mortality: Findings from a Population-based Propensity-matched Analysis," *American Journal of Epidemiology* 178 (2013): 1571-1578.

175 *If you are a grandparent, and not too frail, a great way to foster your health is to babysit your grandkids.* —Sonja Hilbrand et al., "Caregiving within and beyond the family is associated with lower mortality for the caregiver: A prospective study," *Evolution and Human Behavior* 38 (2017): 397-403.

177 *In one such "real" experiment in which university students carried out acts of random kindness over the course of three weeks . . .* —Nicola Catherine Paviglianiti and Jennifer D. Irwin, "Students' Experiences of a Voluntary Random Acts of Kindness Health Promotion Project," *Youth Engagement in Health Promotion* 1 (2017).

177 *In one South California study, participants who were assigned to conduct random acts of kindness . . .* —S. Katherine Nelson-Coffey et al., "Kindness in the blood: A randomized controlled trial of the gene regulatory impact of prosocial behavior," *Psychoneuroendocrinology* 81 (2017): 8-13.

178 *Yet when such patients are asked to write kind letters to people who are awaiting a transplant . . .* —Christine Rini et al., "Harnessing Benefits of Helping Others: A Randomized Controlled Trial Testing Expressive Helping to Address Survivorship Problems After Hematopoietic Stem Cell Transplant," *Health Psychology* 33 (2014): 1541-1551.

178 *"We talked. We knew what was going on there and there was always someone around to help you and to keep you from feeling lonely."* —Bruhn, John G. and Stewart Wolf. *The Roseto Story: An Anatomy of Health* (University of Oklahoma Press, 1979).

179 *In communities with high social cohesion . . .* —Samson Y. Gebreab et al., "Neighborhood social and physical environments and type 2 diabetes mellitus in African Americans: The Jackson Heart Study," *Health & Place* 43 (2017): 128-137.

179 *. . . low social cohesion can mean an increased risk of dying from a heart attack.* —Jan Sundquist et al., "Low linking social capital as a predictor of coronary heart disease in Sweden: A cohort study of 2.8 million people," *Social Science & Medicine* 62 (2006): 954-963.

179 *The effects of such spatial stigma can be seen in New York City . . .* —Duncan, Dustin T. and Ichiro Kawachi. *Neighborhoods and Health* (Oxford, UK: Oxford University Press, 2018).

179 *Studies from places as diverse as the US, Malaysia, and Poland itself show that residents of such gated areas report lower sense of belonging.* —Georjeanna Wilson-Doenges, "An Exploration of Sense of Community and Fear of Crime in Gated Communities," *Environment and Behavior* 32 (2000): 597-611.

181 *"attracted people like moths to a flame."* —Sarah Kobos, "Be a Better Neighbor, Build a Better Neighborhood," Strong Towns, accessed August 8, 2019, https://www.strongtowns.org/journal/2018/4/12/eight-ways-to-be-a-better-neighbor

181 *"Neighbors walked over to see what was going on. People driving by stopped to hang out and chat. Before long, we had to open more wine and bring out the dining room chairs."* —ibid.

181 *Research shows that people who volunteer for self-oriented reasons . . .* —Sara Konrath et al., "Motives for Volunteering Are Associated with Mortality Risk in Older Adults," *Health Psychology* (2011).

182 *A few years back, Lara Aknin's research assistants walked around the campus of the University of British Columbia . . .* —Lara B. Aknin et al., "Making a difference matters: Impact unlocks the emotional benefits of prosocial spending," *Journal of Economic Behavior & Organization* 88 (2013): 90-95.

183 *. . . the reward areas of the brain, the ventral striatum and septal areas, activate more . . .* —William T. Harbaugh, Ulrich Mayr and Daniel R. Burghart, "Neural responses to taxation and voluntary giving reveal motives for charitable donations," *Science* 316 (2007): 1622–1625.

183 *Kids who are promised something in return for volunteering may do the tasks more eagerly at first* . . . —Felix Warneken and Michael Tomasello, "Extrinsic rewards undermine altruistic tendencies in 20-month-olds," *Developmental Psychology*, 44 (2008): 1785-1788.

184 *. . . some studies find top wellness returns for under a hundred hours of volunteering per year, while other claim that number is a mere forty.* —Jane Allyn Piliavin and Erica Siegl, "Health Benefits of Volunteering in the Wisconsin Longitudinal Study," *Journal of Health and Social Behavior* 48 (2007): 450-464.

CHAPTER 9: WHY PERSONALITY AND EMOTIONS MATTER FOR LONGEVITY

187 *"God started my life off well by bestowing upon me a grace of inestimable value . . ."* —Deborah Danner, David Snowdon, and Wallace Friesen, "Positive emotions in early life and longevity: Findings from the nun study," *Journal of Personality and Social Psychology* 80 (2001).

188 *Many decades after Mother Kostka sent her call for autobiographies, three University of Kentucky researchers* . . . —Deborah Danner, David Snowdon and Wallace Friesen, "Positive emotions in early life and longevity: Findings from the nun study," *Journal of Personality and Social Psychology* 80 (2001).

189 *It appears that happiness can add anywhere from four to ten years of life.* —Ed Diener and Micaela Y. Chan, "Happy People Live Longer: Subjective Well-Being Contributes to Health and Longevity," *Applied Psychology: Health and Well-Being* 3 (2011): 1-43.

189 *One particularly well-done British study, in which existential enjoyment was measured every two years for six years in total* . . . —Paola Zaninotto, Jane Wardle and Andrew Steptoe, "Sustained enjoyment of life and mortality at older ages: analysis of the English Longitudinal Study of Ageing," *BMJ* 355 (2016).

190 *In one study that directly compared hedonic and eudaemonic well-being . . .* —Barbara L. Fredrickson et al., "A functional genomic perspective on human well-being," *PNAS* 110 (2013): 13684-13689.

191 *If a ninety-year-old with a clear purpose in life develops Alzheimer's disease . . .* — Patricia A. Boyle et al., "Effect of Purpose in Life on the Relation Between Alzheimer Disease Pathologic Changes on Cognitive Function in Advanced Age," *Archives of General Psychiatry* 69 (2012): 499–505.

191 *. . . when "the excrement hits the air conditioning" . . .* —Vonnegut, Kurt. *Hocus Pocus* (New York: The Berkley Publishing Group, 1990).

191 *In lab experiments, when purposeful people are made to look at disgusting or disturbing pictures of violence and sickness . . .* —Carien M. van Reekum et al., "Individual Differences in Amygdala and Ventromedial Prefrontal Cortex Activity are Associated with Evaluation Speed and Psychological Well-being," *Journal of Cognitive Neuroscience* 19 (2007): 237-248.

191 *Besides, eudaemonic well-being means more grey matter in the insula—the reward-related brain area . . .* —Carol D. Ryff et al., "Purposeful Engagement, Healthy Aging, and the Brain," *Current Behavioral Neuroscience Reports* 3 (2016): 318-327.

192 *The more people tend to focus on their financial goals, the less happy they become . . .* —Richard M. Ryan and Edward L. Deci, "On Happiness and Human Potentials: A Review of Research on Hedonic and Eudaimonic Well-Being," *Annual Review of Psychology* 52 (2001): 141–166.

192 *As Ralph Waldo Emerson once wrote, "Want is a growing giant whom the coat of Have was never large enough to cover."* —Emerson, Ralph Waldo. *The Prose Works of Ralph Waldo Emerson, Volume 2* (Boston; James R. Osgood and Company, 1876), 377.

193 *It was nighttime. A single lab rat entered his experimental outdoor pen . . .* —M. Berdoy, J. P. Webster and D. W. Macdonald, "Fatal attraction in rats infected with Toxoplasma gondii," *Proceedings of The Royal Society* B 267 (2000): 1591-1594.

194 *. . . once this tiny parasite makes its home in a person's body, that person could become more impulsive, sensation-seeking, and aggressive . . .* —Victor Otero Martinez et al., "*Toxoplasma gondii* infection and behavioral outcomes in humans: a systematic review," *Parasitology Research* 117 (2018): 3059-3065.

194 *. . . (there are even some initial suggestions that T. gondii increases the risk of having traffic accidents) . . .* —Shaban Gohardehi et al., "The potential risk of toxoplasmosis for traffic accidents: A systematic review and meta-analysis," *Experimental Parasitology* 191 (2018): 19-24.

194 *Bolder, more aggressive trout have shorter telomeres in their fins . . .* —Bart Adriaenssens et al., "Telomere length covaries with personality in wild brown trout," *Physiology & Behavior* 165 (2016): 217-222.

194 *In people, the connection between personality and health is already so well established that some researchers . . .* —Benjamin P. Chapman, Brent Roberts and Paul Duberstein, "Personality and Longevity: Knowns, Unknowns, and Implications for Public Health and Personalized Medicine," *Journal of Aging Research* (2011).

195 *The positive effects of being organized and industrious are found all across the planet . . .* —Margaret L. Kern and Howard S. Friedman, "Do Conscientious Individuals Live Longer? A Quantitative Review," *Health Psychology* 27 (2008): 505-512.

195 *Conscientiousness measured in childhood can predict longevity even as far as seven decades into the future.* —Howard S. Friedman et al., "Does Childhood Personality Predict Longevity?" *Journal of Personality and Social Psychology* 65 (1993): 176-185.

196 *If the above seems to describe you, you may be in trouble, since being neurotic can mean even 33 percent higher risk of mortality.* —Robert S. Wilson et al., "Neuroticism, Extraversion, and Mortality in a Defined Population of Older Persons," *Psychosomatic Medicine* 67 (2005): 841–845.

196 *In the Netherlands, for instance, the top most neurotic people cost the country over $1.3 billion per year per million inhabitants in health services, out-of-pocket costs, and production losses.* —Pim Cuijpers et al., "Economic Costs of Neuroticism: A Population-Based Study," *JAMA Psychiatry* (2010).

196 *. . . the most neurotic countries — that would be Greece, followed by Russia . . .* — Richard Lynn and Terence Martin, "National differences for thirty-seven nations

in extraversion, neuroticism, psychoticism and economic, demographic and other correlates," *Personality and Individual Differences* 19 (1995): 403-406.

196 *In the US, Pennsylvania, Ohio, and New York have the most neurotic people, while Alaska and Arizona have the least.* —Peter Jason Rentfrow, "Statewide Differences in Personality," *American Psychologist* 65 (2010): 548-558.

197 *People who worry a lot tend to have fewer natural killer cells—lymphocytes that launch attacks against infections and tumours.* —Suzanne C. Segerstrom et al., "Relationship of Worry to Immune Sequelae of the Northridge Earthquake," *Journal of Behavioral Medicine* 21 (1998): 433-450.

197 *. . . worry-prone men who have suffered a myocardial infarction are more likely to get unlucky a second time.* —Laura D. Kubzansky et al., "Is worrying bad for your heart? A prospective study of worry and coronary heart disease in the normative aging study," *Circulation* 95 (1997): 818–824.

197 *In one study, patients with hernias who fretted about the procedure the most . . .* —Elizabeth Broadbent et al., "Psychological Stress Impairs Early Wound Repair Following Surgery," *Psychosomatic Medicine* 65 (2003): 865-869.

197 *. . . follow-up studies haven't confirmed the effects of type A personality on heart attacks or clogged arteries.* —David R. Ragland and Richard J. Brand, "Type A Behavior and Mortality from Coronary Heart Disease," *The New England Journal of Medicine* 318 (1988): 65-60.

197 *In recent years, it came to light that the tobacco industry . . .* —Mark P. Petticrew, Kelley Lee and Martin McKee, "Type A Behavior Pattern and Coronary Heart Disease: Philip Morris's 'Crown Jewel,' *American Journal of Public Health* 102 (2012): 2018-2025.

198 *It can cause problems with your triglycerides, your glucose levels, and your insulin resistance.* —Loren L. Toussaint et al., "Hostility, Forgiveness, and Cognitive Impairment Over 10 Years in a National Sample of American Adults," *Health Psychology* 37 (2018): 1102-1106.

198 *. . . hostility is particularly detrimental to women, messing with the inflammatory processes in their bodies . . .* —Julie Boisclair Demarble et al., "The relation between hostility and concurrent levels of inflammation is sex, age, and measure dependent," *Journal of Psychosomatic Research* 76 (2014): 384-393.

198 *They have shorter telomeres, and their inflammatory proteins are as elevated as if they were ten years older than they really are.* —D. Schoormans et al., "Leukocyte telomere length and personality: associations with the Big Five and Type D personality traits," *Psychological Medicine* 48 (2018): 1008-1019.

198 *Type Ds are also prone to having something called "soft" or "vulnerable" plaque, which is a perfect recipe for a heart attack.* —Nina Kupper and Johan Denollet, "Type D Personality as a Risk Factor in Coronary Heart Disease: a Review of Current Evidence," *Current Cardiology Reports* 20 (2018).

199 *They are also almost four times more likely to die than other patients with coronary heart disease.* —ibid.

199 *Human nature tends to shift with age toward less neurotic, less extroverted, and less open to experience but more agreeable.* —William J. Chopik and Shinobu Kitayama, "Personality change across the life span: Insights from a cross-cultural, longitudinal study," *Journal of Personality* 86 (2018): 508-521.

199 *One study done on over three hundred spouses living in Florida . . .* —Justin A. Lavner et al., "Personality Change among Newlyweds: Patterns, Predictors, and Associations with Marital Satisfaction over Time," *Developmental Psychology* 54 (2018): 1172-1185.

200 *There are some reports that divorce increases extraversion in women . . .* —Paul T. Costa, Jr. et al., "Personality at Midlife: Stability, Intrinsic Maturation, and Response to Life Events," *Assessment* 7 (2000): 365-378.

200 *. . . and joining the military can make you less agreeable.* —Joshua J. Jackson et al., "Military training and personality trait development: Does the military make the man, or does the man make the military?" *Psychological Science* 23 (2012): 270–277.

200 *Some personality dimensions are harder to budge, such as openness to experience. Neuroticism, meanwhile, is the easiest trait to work on . . .* —Brent W. Roberts et al., "A Systematic Review of Personality Trait Change Through Intervention," *Psychological Bulletin* (2017).

200 *In one particularly thorough study, close to four hundred students from the University of Illinois at Urbana-Champaign and Michigan State University . . .* —Nathan W. Hudson et al., "You have to follow through: Attaining behavioral change goals predicts volitional personality change," *Journal of Personality and Social Psychology* (2018).

202 *Their active compound, psilocybin, has been shown to shift certain personality dimensions even after a single dose . . .* —Katherine A. MacLean, Matthew W. Johnson and Roland R. Griffiths, "Mystical Experiences Occasioned by the Hallucinogen Psilocybin Lead to Increases in the Personality Domain of Openness," *Journal of Psychopharmacology* 25 (2011): 1453–1461.

202 *A study of over a thousand American veterans suggested that Mr. Sulky may be in for trouble . . .* —Daniel K. Mroczek and Avron Spiro, III, "Personality Change Influences Mortality in Older Men," *Psychological Science* 18 (2007): 371–376.

202 *Some emerging research is beginning to indicate that helicopter parenting may lead to neuroticism . . .* —Chris Segrin et al., "Parent and Child Traits Associated with Overparenting," *Journal of Social and Clinical Psychology* 32 (2013): 569-595.

CHAPTER 10: HOW MEDITATION AND MINDFULNESS BOOST HEALTH

206 *"The meditation buzz is incredible," Harrison claimed in one interview. "I get higher than I ever did with drugs."* —David Chiu, "The Beatles in India: 16 Things You Didn't Know," *Rolling Stone*, accessed August 8, 2019, https://www.rollingstone.com/music/music-news/the-beatles-in-india-16-things-you-didnt-know-203601/

208 *In one 2018 experiment, just one month spent at Spirit Rock Meditation Center in Woodacre, California . . .* —Quinn A. Conklin et al., "Insight meditation and

telomere biology: The effects of intensive retreat and the moderating role of personality, " *Brain, Behavior, and Immunity* 70 (2018): 233-245.

208 *Expert Zen meditators who have practiced daily for over ten years . . .* —Marta Alda et al., "Zen meditation, Length of Telomeres, and the Role of Experiential Avoidance and Compassion," *Mindfulness* 7 (2016): 651-659.

208 *DNA from the blood cells of long-term meditators show changes suggesting that the more you practise, the more slowly you age.* —Raphaëlle Chaix et al., "Epigenetic clock analysis in long-term meditators," *Psychoneuroendocrinology* 85 (2017): 210-214.

208 *And even though staying at hippie California retreats may not necessarily rebalance your chakras, it may change your FOXO genes . . .* —E.S. Epel, "Meditation and vacation effects have an impact on disease-associated molecular phenotypes," *Translational Psychiatry* 6 (2016).

208 *If you put someone who meditates a lot into a neuroimaging machine . . .* —Yi-Yuan Tang, Britta K. Hölzel and Michael I. Posner, "The neuroscience of mindfulness meditation," *Nature Reviews Neuroscience* 16 (2015): 213-225.

209 *A typical meditation expert, meanwhile, will have a particularly large hippocampus compared to an average Joe . . .* —B. Rael Cahn et al., "Yoga, Meditation and Mind-Body Health: Increased BDNF, Cortisol Awakening Response, and Altered Inflammatory Marker Expression after a 3-Month Yoga and Meditation Retreat," *Frontiers in Human Neuroscience* (2017).

209 *Volunteers participating in a three-month yoga and meditation retreat saw their plasma levels of BDNF triple . . .* —B. Rael Cahn et al., "Yoga, Meditation and Mind-Body Health: Increased BDNF, Cortisol Awakening Response, and Altered Inflammatory Marker Expression after a 3-Month Yoga and Meditation Retreat," *Frontiers in Human Neuroscience* (2017).

210 *When a group of students watched the 1974 version of The Texas Chainsaw Massacre . . .* —Rubina Mian, Graeme McLaren and David W. Macdonald, "Of Stress, Mice and Men: a Radical Approach to Old Problems," in *Stress and Health: New Research,* ed. Kimberly V. Oxington (New York: Nova Science Publications, 2005), 61-79.

212 *Take the one done at the University of Wisconsin-Madison that involved sixty-eight volunteers.* —Melissa A. Rosenkranz et al., "Reduced stress and inflammatory responsiveness in experienced meditators compared to a matched healthy control group," *Psychoneuroendocrinology* 68 (2016): 117-125.

213 *. . . even after just a few weeks of meditation, you can see reduced expression of pro-inflammatory genes in white blood cells.* —Ivana Buric et al., "What Is the Molecular Signature of Mind–Body Interventions? A Systematic Review of Gene Expression Changes Induced by Meditation and Related Practices," *Frontiers in Immunology* (2017).

213 *Experiments with the flu vaccine confirm that this can help produce higher antibody titres . . .* —Bret Stetka, "Changing Our DNA through Mind Control?" *Scientific American,* accessed August 8, 2019, https://www.scientificamerican.com/article/changing-our-dna-through-mind-control/

213 *In one experiment, volunteers had to rate how much it hurt them when researchers applied a pad heated to 120 degrees Fahrenheit (49°C) to their leg . . .* —Fadel Zeidan et al., "Mindfulness Meditation-Based Pain Relief Employs Different Neural Mechanisms Than Placebo and Sham Mindfulness Meditation-Induced Analgesia," *Journal of Neuroscience* 35 (2015): 15307-15325.

214 *When people with lots of meditation experience go for an intense, one-day retreat . . .* —Perla Kaliman et al., "Rapid changes in histone deacetylases and inflammatory gene expression in expert meditators," *Psychoneuroendocrinology* 40 (2014): 96-107.

214 *For now, the authors of a 2016 review published in the prestigious* Annals of the New York Academy of Sciences *. . .* —David S. Black and George M. Slavich, "Mindfulness meditation and the immune system: a systematic review of randomized controlled trials," *Annals of the New York Academy of Sciences* 1373 (2016): 13-24.

215 *"We still see and hear the water, but we are out of the torrent."* —Kabat-Zinn, Jon. *Wherever You Go, There You Are: Mindfulness Meditation in Everyday Life* (New York: Hyperion Books, 2005), 94.

216 *Studies confirm that greater levels of mindfulness correlate to greater satisfaction in romantic relationships.* —Johan C. Karremans, Melanie P. J. Schellekens and Gesa Kappen, "Bridging the Sciences of Mindfulness and Romantic Relationships: A Theoretical Model and Research Agenda," *Personality and Social Psychology Review* 21 (2017): 29-49.

216 *. . . eight-week-long mindfulness programs can increase relationship satisfaction.* —James W. Carson et al., "Mindfulness-Based Relationship Enhancement," *Behavior Therapy* 35 (2004): 471-494.

216 *Some psychologists suggest that meditation may work only for committed relationships . . .* —Johan C. Karremans, Melanie P. J. Schellekens and Gesa Kappen, "Bridging the Sciences of Mindfulness and Romantic Relationships: A Theoretical Model and Research Agenda," *Personality and Social Psychology Review* 21 (2017): 29-49.

217 *"When I enter her room now, I can feel myself soften."* —James W. Carson et al., "Loving-Kindness Meditation for Chronic Low Back Pain," *Journal of Holistic Nursing* 23 (2005): 287-304.

217 *After two weeks of loving-kindness meditation, people are willing to donate almost twice as much money . . .* —Helen Y. Weng et al., "Compassion training alters altruism and neural responses to suffering," *Psychological Science* 24 (2013): 1171-1180.

218 *They did indeed conclude that students who, for two and a half months, wrote down five things per week they could be thankful for . . .* —Emmons and Michael E. McCullough, "Counting Blessings Versus Burdens: An Experimental Investigation of Gratitude and Subjective Well-Being in Daily Life," *Journal of Personality and Social Psychology* 84 (2003): 377-389.

218 *A 2017 review of thirty-eight studies concluded that . . .* —Leah R. Dickens, "Using Gratitude to Promote Positive Change: A Series of Meta-Analyses Investigating

the Effectiveness of Gratitude Interventions," *Basic and Applied Social Psychology* 39 (2017): 193-208.

221   *The review concluded that "yoga interventions appear to be equal or superior to exercise in nearly every outcome measured except those involving physical fitness."* —Alyson Ross and Sue Thomas, "The Health Benefits of Yoga and Exercise: A Review of Comparison Studies," *Journal of Alternative and Complementary Medicine* 16 (2010): 3-12.

221   *. . . for patients with fibromyalgia, yoga can bring greater relief of symptoms than FDA-recommended drug therapies.* —James W. Carson et al., "A pilot randomized controlled trial of the Yoga of Awareness program in the management of fibromyalgia," *Pain* 151 (2010): 530-539.

221   *A curious series of experiments involving albino rats . . .* —Donald J. Noble et al., "Slow Breathing Can Be Operantly Conditioned in the Rat and May Reduce Sensitivity to Experimental Stressors," *Frontiers in Physiology* (2017).

222   *While at rest, long-term practitioners of mindful meditation inhale and exhale fewer times per minute than your typical human.* —Joseph Wielgosz et al., "Long-term mindfulness training is associated with reliable differences in resting respiration rate," *Scientific Reports* 6 (2016).

222   *They also blink less and in a different pattern.* —Ayla Kruis et al., "Effects of Meditation Practice on Spontaneous Eye Blink Rate," *Psychophysiology* 53 (2016): 749-758.

223   *Even though the activity of the enzyme that protects the tips of chromosomes, telomerase, can increase after just a few weeks . . .* —Cecile A. Lengacher et al., "Influence of Mindfulness-Based Stress Reduction (MBSR) on Telomerase Activity in Women With Breast Cancer (BC)," *Biological Research for Nursing* 16 (2014): 438-447.

223   *Kabat-Zinn once wrote, "Five minutes of formal practice can be as profound or more so than forty-five minutes . . ."* —Kabat-Zinn, Jon. *Wherever You Go, There You Are: Mindfulness Meditation in Everyday Life* (New York: Hyperion Books, 2005).

224   *One such comparison based on over three hundred trials, which included an astounding fifty-three yoga types . . .* —Holger Cramer et al., "Is one yoga style better than another? A systematic review of associations of yoga style and conclusions in randomized yoga trials," *Complementary Therapies in Medicine* 25 (2016): 178-187.

224   *If you want to reduce your risk of cardiovascular disease, for instance, transcendental meditation may be a particularly good idea.* —Robert H. Schneider, Jeremy Z. Fields and John Salerno, "Editorial commentary on AHA scientiflc statement on meditation and cardiovascular risk reduction," *Journal of the American Society of Hypertension* (2018): 1-2.

224   *. . . tai chi has been linked to the reduction of severity of fibromyalgia . . .* —Chenchen Wang et al., "A Randomized Trial of Tai Chi for Fibromyalgia," *New England Journal of Medicine* 363 (2010): 743-754.

224 *. . . qigong may help with fatigue and boost the activity of telomerase.* —Rainbow T. H. Ho et al., "A Randomized Controlled Trial of Qigong Exercise on Fatigue Symptoms, Functioning, and Telomerase Activity in Persons with Chronic Fatigue or Chronic Fatigue Syndrome," *Annals of Behavioral Medicine* 44 (2012): 160-170.

CHAPTER 11: LONGEVITY LESSONS FROM JAPAN

229 *Among Japanese men age forty-five to fifty-four, over 70 percent have some form of checkup at least once per year.* —Nayu Ikeda et al., "What has made the population of Japan healthy? " *The Lancet* 378 (2011): 1094-1105.

230 *Carriers of the ApoE4 allele, many of whom are of Scandinavian decent, are at about 40 percent higher risk of a heart disease . . .* —Caleb E. Finch, "Evolution of the Human Lifespan and Diseases of Aging: Roles of Infection, Inflammation, and Nutrition," *PNAS* 107 (2010): 1718-1724.

230 *For example, generally shortish Greeks and Italians who move to Australia tend to out-live the taller locals by about four years.* —Thomas T. Samaras and Harold Elrick, "Height, body size, and longevity: is smaller better for the human body?" *Western Journal of Medicine* 176 (2002): 206-208.

231 *When the Japanese relocate to California, rates of heart disease among them double.* —M.G. Marmot et al., "Epidemiologic studies of coronary heart disease and stroke in Japanese men living in Japan, Hawaii and California: prevalence of coronary and hypertensive heart disease and associated risk factors," *American Journal of Epidemiology* 102 (1975).

232 *. . . they down 27 percent more greens than does an average Yamada Tarō.* —"Asian Parliamentarians' Study Visit on Population and Development: Aging in Japan—Tokyo and Nagano," The Asian Population and Development Association, accessed August 10, 2019, http://www.apda.jp/pdf/p02_report/2015_Meeting_Minutes-Study_Visit-Aging_in_Japan_en.pdf

233 *As De Tocqueville once said, "Such folk owe no man anything and hardly expect any-thing from anybody."* —de Tocqueville, Alexis. *Democracy in America* (Chicago: University of Chicago Press, 2000).

234 *Some researchers believe that Japan's collectivism may have its roots in the way rice is grown.* —Shiro Horiuchi, "Major Causes of the Rapid Longevity Extension in Postwar Japan," *The Japanese Journal of Population* 9 (2011).

236 *According to one study, going to such a centre even once a week lowers the risk of develop-ing dementia by 40 percent.* —Hui-Xin Wang, Anita Karp, Bengt Winblad, and Laura Fratiglioni, "Late-life engagement in social and leisure activities is asso-ciated with a decreased risk of dementia: A longitudinal study from the Kungsholmen project," *American Journal of Epidemiology* 155 (2002): 1081-108.

236 *If each and every older adult in Canada picked up one social activity . . .* —Sheila Novek et al., "Exploring the Impacts of Senior Centres on Older Adults," The Centre on Aging, University of Manitoba, accessed August 10, 2019, https://www.gov.mb.ca/seniors/publications/docs/senior_centre_report.pdf

237 *. . . so much so that by the 1990s, over 90 percent of the people here considered themselves to be middle class.* —Nayu Ikeda et al., "What has made the population of Japan healthy?" *The Lancet* 378 (2011): 1094-1105.

237 *One meta-analysis of studies conducted in eleven countries including Japan, Canada, and the US . . .* —Naoki Kondo et al., "Income inequality, mortality, and self rated health: meta-analysis of multilevel studies," *BMJ* 339 (2009).

239 *In one longitudinal survey, those seventy-five-year-olds who worked a paid job over a hundred hours a year in 1998 . . .* —Ming-Ching Luoh and A. Regula Herzog, "Individual Consequences of Volunteer and Paid Work in Old Age: Health and Mortality," *Journal of Health and Social Behavior* 43 (2002): 490-509.

240 *Japan scored the highest in terms of the percentage of people who answered "very much" to these claims . . .* —Yoosung Park et al., "Sense of "ikigai" (reason for living) and social support in the Asia-Pacific region," *Behaviormetrika* 42 (2015): 191-208.

240 *In a study that followed over forty thousand Japanese for seven years, among people who had ikigai at day one . . .* —Toshimasa Sona, "Sense of Life Worth Living (*Ikigai*) and Mortality in Japan: Ohsaki Study," *Psychosomatic Medicine* 70 (2008): 709-715.

242 *"After studying to be a Zen teacher for many years, Teno went to visit Nan-in, an old Zen master.* —Reps, Paul and Nyogen Senzaki, *Zen Flesh, Zen Bones: A Collection of Zen and Pre-Zen Writings* (North Clarendon: Tuttle Publishing, 1957), cited in: Steve John Powell, "The Japanese skill copied by the world," BBC, accessed August 11, 2019, http://www.bbc.com/travel/story/20170504-the-japanese-skill-copied-by-the-world

243 *. . . Zen meditation experts have longer telomeres than those who don't follow the practice.* —Marta Alda et al., "Zen meditation, Length of Telomeres, and the Role of Experiential Avoidance and Compassion," *Mindfulness* 7 (2016): 651-659.

243 *Zen meditation also increases heart rate variability and helps with pain.* —Caroline Peressutti et al., "Heart rate dynamics in different levels of Zen meditation," *International Journal of Cardiology* 145 (2010): 142-146 AND Joshua A. Grant, Jérôme Courtemanche and Pierre Rainville, "A non-elaborative mental stance and decoupling of executive and pain-related cortices predicts low pain sensitivity in Zen meditators," *Pain* 152 (2011): 150-156.

EPILOGUE

247 *"Eat food. Not too much. Mostly plants . . ."* —Pollan, Michael, "Unhappy Meals," *The New York Times*, accessed October 8, 2019, https://www.nytimes.com/2007/01/28/magazine/28nutritionism.t.html

More notes and resources can be found at
www.GrowingYoungTheBook.com

INDEX